W9-BLR-839

The TYPE 2
DIABETIC
COOKBOOK
AND ACTION PLAN

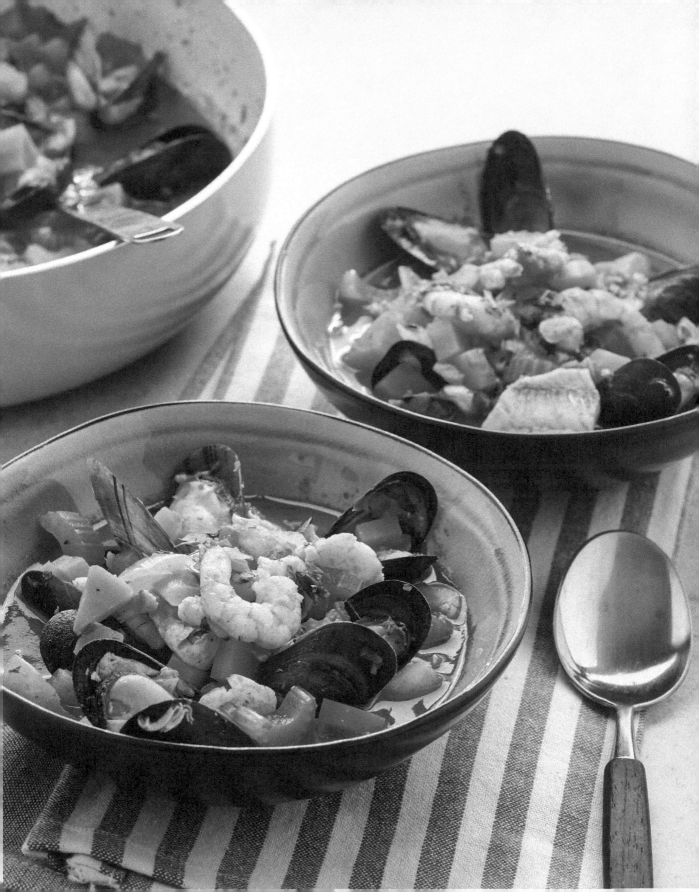

The TYPE 2 DIABETIC COOKBOOK

AND ACTION PLAN

A THREE-MONTH KICKSTART GUIDE for LIVING WELL with TYPE 2 DIABETES

MARTHA MCKITTRICK, RDN, CDE

MICHELLE ANDERSON

Copyright © 2017 by Martha McKittrick

No part of this publication may be reproduced, stored in a retrieval system, or transmitted in any form or by any means, electronic, mechanical, photocopying, recording, scanning or otherwise, except as permitted under Section 107 or 108 of the 1976 United States Copyright Act, without the prior written permission of the publisher. Requests to the publisher for permission should be addressed to the Permissions Department, Rockridge Press, 6001 Shellmound St., Suite 175, Emeryville, CA, 94608.

Limit of Liability/Disclaimer of Warranty: The publisher and the author make no representations or warranties with respect to the accuracy or completeness of the contents of this work and specifically disclaim all warranties, including without limitation warranties of fitness for a particular purpose. No warranty may be created or extended by sales or promotional materials. The advice and strategies contained herein may not be suitable for every situation. This work is sold with the understanding that the publisher is not engaged in rendering medical, legal, or other professional advice or services. If professional assistance is required, the services of a competent professional person should be sought. Neither the publisher nor the author shall be liable for damages arising herefrom. The fact that an individual, organization, or website is referred to in this work as a citation and/or potential source of further information does not mean that the author or the publisher endorses the information the individual, organization, or website may provide or recommendations they/it may make. Further, readers should be aware that Internet websites listed in this work may have changed or disappeared between when this work was written and when it is read.

For general information on our other products and services or to obtain technical support, please contact our Customer Care Department within the United States at (866) 744-2665, or outside the United States at (510) 253-0500.

Rockridge Press publishes its books in a variety of electronic and print formats. Some content that appears in print may not be available in electronic books, and vice versa.

TRADEMARKS: Rockridge Press and the Rockridge Press logo are trademarks or registered trademarks of Callisto Media Inc. and/or its affiliates, in the United States and other countries, and may not be used without written permission. All other trademarks are the property of their respective owners. Rockridge Press is not associated with any product or vendor mentioned in this book.

Cover design by Kathleen Lynch

Interior photography: © Darren Muir (photos) & Yolanda Muir (food styling), pp. 2, 42, 86, 114, 128, 142, 154, 166, 188, 202; Stockfood/Sarka Babicka, p.6; Stockfood/Claudia Timmann, p.12; Stocksy/Laura Adani, p.32; Front cover photography: StockFood/People Pictures; Back cover photography: Stockfood/People Pictures, Stockfood/People Pictures, Stockfood/Alan Richardson

ISBN: Print 978-1-62315-833-0 | eBook 978-1-62315-834-7

R1

To everyone living with diabetes

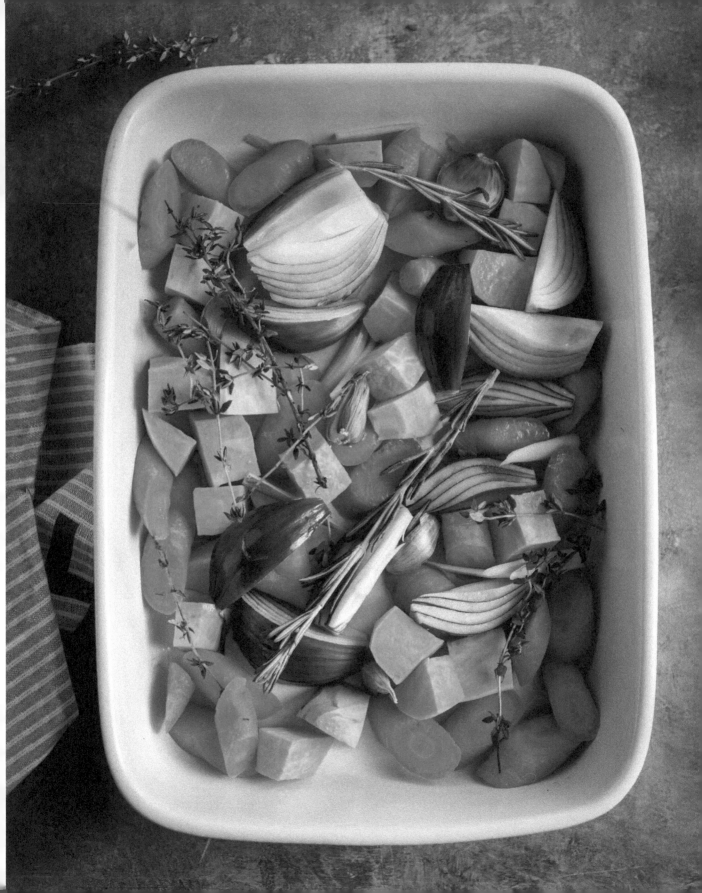

CONTENTS

PART 2: THE RECIPES

INTRODUCTION

A diagnosis of diabetes can be frightening. You may be in a state of shock and vaguely hear your doctor talk about blood sugar numbers, blood testing, medications, and potential complications. For many people, their thoughts immediately turn to food. After all, eating is one of life's greatest pleasures. As a certified diabetes educator, the first questions my patients usually ask me are, "What can I eat? Will I have to cut out my favorite foods? Are bread, pasta, and sweets off-limits forever? How will I cook for my family if I have to be on a special diet?"

The changes you have to make might feel overwhelming. Conflicting advice from friends and the media can make things even more confusing. But here's the good news: Type 2 diabetes is manageable. Best of all, you will still be able to eat your favorite foods. And yes, that does include bread, pasta, and sweets—in moderation, of course! *The Type 2 Diabetic Cookbook and Action Plan* is here to help you. We will give you step-by-step guidance on tackling the diet and lifestyle changes that can help you manage type 2 diabetes. So . . . take a deep breath and read on.

The main goal of type 2 diabetes treatment is to effectively manage your blood sugar through food choices and physical activity. Good blood sugar control is important in order to help prevent complications. While some people may need medications, the good news is that many people can manage their diabetes with lifestyle changes alone. That includes losing weight if you are overweight, exercising regularly, and eating a healthy diet.

In the past, diabetic diets were very restrictive. Thirty years ago, when I first started counseling patients with diabetes, I remember advising them to avoid sugar and all desserts and to follow a rigid "exchange" type plan. Food was divided into six different groups, or exchange lists. Each exchange list contained foods with about the same amount of carbohydrate, protein, fat, and calories. For example, for breakfast you might be allowed one fruit exchange, two bread exchanges, one milk exchange, one meat exchange, and one fat exchange. While this system can be helpful for meal planning, it can also be somewhat inflexible.

But times have changed! While you will probably need to make some changes in what you are eating, you will have the flexibility to include the foods you enjoy. Adjusting to a new relationship with food can be challenging, and we're here for you every step of the way. We want to make it easy, so you don't feel overwhelmed. That's why we've taken the guesswork out of what to eat to manage your diabetes.

Here is what you will find in this book as we guide you through the first three months:

Month 1: Learn the basics of a healthy diet and how foods affect your blood sugar and overall health. Get the lowdown on carbohydrate counting and the glycemic index/load. Best of all, use the very clear instructions for two weeks of meal plans—including detailed shopping lists.

Month 2: Focus on physical activity and stress management, as they play key roles in blood sugar management. Get more details on nutrition, mindful eating, and weight-loss tips. Stock your kitchen and get ready to prepare diabetes-friendly meals.

Month 3: Get practical tips for dealing with diabetes mentally and emotionally. The tips include guidance for social situations, dining out, and troubling moments, as well as other support.

When you have type 2 diabetes, you become a member of a team. Your doctor, nurse, dietitian, certified diabetes educator, pharmacist, psychologist, podiatrist, and other specialists are all working to help you. It's important that you discuss with your team your treatment goals and how to achieve them. Diabetes is not a one-size-fits-all condition, and you need a care plan tailored for you.

Diabetes is not a doomsday diagnosis. On the contrary, I've had many patients tell me that getting diagnosed helped them take better care of themselves. They've lost weight and feel more energetic and healthier overall. Play an active role in your own health and take charge of your diabetes!

PART ONE

Getting Started

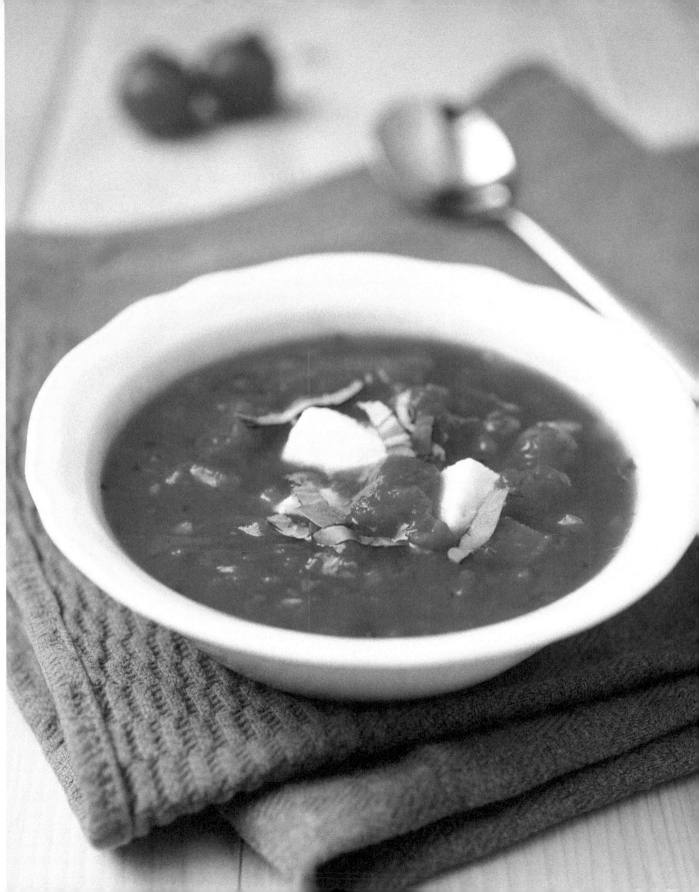

CHAPTER 1

Understanding Type 2 Diabetes

If you've been diagnosed with diabetes, you aren't alone. In 2014, the U.S. Centers for Disease Control and Prevention called diabetes an "emerging epidemic." An estimated 9.3 percent of the population—29.1 million Americans—have diabetes. Of them, 90 to 95 percent have type 2 diabetes. And it's estimated that as many as one in three American adults will have diabetes by 2050, if the current trends continue.

You may be wondering why you got diabetes. The exact cause isn't known, but there are several risk factors, including genetics, physical inactivity, prediabetes, gestational diabetes (GDM), family history, race and ethnicity, age, high blood pressure, and abnormal cholesterol. But the biggest risk factor for type 2 diabetes is being overweight or obese. As the rates of obesity in our nation skyrocket, so do the rates of type 2 diabetes. Seventy percent of Americans are obese or overweight, as compared to 60 percent ten years ago.

It's no wonder we are gaining weight, because we live in an "obeseogenic" environment. We sit more, move less, work longer hours, and are more dependent on technology. The availability of fast food, how often we eat out, the overabundance of highly processed foods, and the supersizing of food portions are major factors in our expanding waistlines. Research done by Lisa Young, PhD, RD, revealed that many restaurant portions are two to five times larger than they were 20 years ago.

And it's not just more calories. The standard American diet is loaded with unhealthy fats, sugar, highly processed carbohydrates, and sodium and is low in fruits, vegetables, and whole grains. Our obeseogenic environment and poor-quality diets affect our weight, risk of diabetes, and overall blood sugar control.

So are we doomed to be overweight and have poor blood sugar control? Absolutely not! Awareness is step number one. Diet plays a major role in controlling blood sugar and promoting weight loss. Let's start with a little understanding of how food works in the body. Then get ready for some easy, healthy, and tasty recipes!

What Is Diabetes?

Diabetes is a condition where the body is no longer able to self-regulate blood glucose. When you eat a food that contains carbohydrate—whether it comes from honey, an apple, or brown rice—the body breaks it down into sugar (also called glucose) during digestion. This glucose passes through the walls of the intestines into the blood, which causes blood sugar (the amount of glucose circulating in the blood) to rise.

In response, the pancreas secretes a hormone called insulin. The role of insulin is to lower the blood sugar back to normal levels. It does this by moving the sugar out of the blood and into the cells, where it is used for energy. Think of insulin as a key that unlocks the doors to the cells. But if you have diabetes, either the body doesn't make enough insulin or the cells don't respond to the insulin. This causes the blood sugar to build up in the bloodstream, resulting in high blood sugar.

Type 2 diabetes usually begins with insulin resistance. The muscle, fat, and liver cells no longer respond to insulin, so the pancreas secretes large amounts of it, trying to keep blood sugar levels within a normal range. Being overweight and physically inactive contributes further to insulin resistance.

Insulin resistance is also found in prediabetes or glucose intolerance. An estimated 79 million Americans have prediabetes. I tell my patients that prediabetes is a warning bell to take action to help prevent diabetes. Studies have shown that losing 7 percent of your body weight, along with regular exercise, can decrease the risk of type 2 diabetes by 58 percent. Once you have diabetes, losing weight, regular exercise, eating carbohydrates in moderation, and maintaining a healthy diet can decrease insulin resistance. This, in turn, will promote better blood sugar control.

A diabetes diagnosis means that the pancreas is not able to produce enough insulin to keep up with this resistance—and insulin deficiency is the result. If your body can't make enough insulin, blood sugar levels become elevated. Long-term elevated blood sugar levels can affect almost every system in the body. Health complications can include heart disease, stroke, kidney failure, nerve damage, eye damage, and blindness. This is why it is so important to work with your health-care team to come up with the best treatment plan for you, and for you to take the leading part in your plan by eating healthy, staying physically active, and losing weight if necessary.

What's the Difference?

	TYPE 1	TYPE 2
Who it affects	Accounts for 5 to 10 percent of all cases of diabetes. It was once called "juvenile onset" diabetes because it was thought to develop most often in children and young adults. We now know it can occur in people of any age, including older adults.	Accounts for 90 to 95 percent of all diagnosed cases of diabetes. It used to be called "adult onset" diabetes, but it is now known that even children— mainly if they're overweight—can develop type 2 diabetes.
What happens	The pancreas makes little if any insulin.	The pancreas doesn't produce enough insulin or the body doesn't respond properly to the insulin that is produced.
Risk factors	Less well-defined, but autoimmune, genetic, and environmental factors are believed to be involved.	Older age, obesity, family history of diabetes, prior history of gestational diabetes, impaired glucose tolerance, physical inactivity, and race/ethnicity.
Treatment	Individualized meal plans, insulin therapy (usually several injections a day), self-monitoring glucose testing several times a day, regular physical activity, and a healthy diet.	A healthy diet, weight loss (if overweight), regular exercise, and monitoring blood glucose levels. Some people are able to manage blood sugar through diet and exercise alone. However, diabetes tends to be a progressive disease, so oral medications and possibly insulin may be needed at some point.

What Is a Healthy Diet for Someone with Diabetes?

People with diabetes often think they need to become strictly focused on avoiding sugar or carbohydrates, and neglect to consider the nutritional quality of their diet. While it's true that carbohydrates have the greatest impact on blood sugar, it is the diet as a whole that contributes to health, weight management, and blood sugar control. Strictly limiting carbohydrates found in fruit and whole grains while eating a diet high in saturated fat and sodium will not promote optimal health.

The American Diabetes Association, the Academy of Nutrition and Dietetics, the American Heart Association, as well as the 2016 New Dietary Guidelines for Americans all emphasize the whole diet, rather than a particular nutrient. It is especially important to follow a heart-healthy diet because your risk for heart disease can be four times greater when you have type 2 diabetes. Cardiovascular disease is the number one cause of illness and death in people with type 2 diabetes.

Focusing on healthy foods, portion control of carbohydrates, and losing weight if you are overweight are the three most important things you can do to manage type 2 diabetes from a nutritional standpoint. And do not feel that you have to get to an unrealistically low weight—even losing 5 to 7 percent of your body weight can help lower blood sugar and reduce the need for diabetic medications. While the exact recommended servings will vary from person to person, here are some guidelines for a healthy diet:

 ◆ Eat a variety of fruits and vegetables.

 ◆ Include whole grains.

 ◆ Aim for two or three servings of fish a week.

 ◆ Include heart-healthy fats such as olive oil, canola oil, nuts and nut butters, seeds, and avocado.

 ◆ Consume fewer than 2,300 milligrams of sodium per day.

 ◆ Limit your intake of added sugars, which are found in sweetened beverages and many processed foods.

Understanding Nutrients

Think of your body like a car: You want to fill it up with quality fuel to make sure it runs optimally. If you have type 2 diabetes, feeding your body with healthy nutrients will help control blood sugar, aid with weight management, decrease your risk of complications, and promote overall health. So here is a crash course in nutrition.

Carbohydrates, proteins, and fats are the three macronutrients your body needs. Carbohydrates have the most significant impact on blood sugar levels. Fats and protein have little or no effect on blood sugar.

PROTEIN

Protein is used for building and repairing tissues, as well as making enzymes, hormones, and other body chemicals. It can also help make you feel more full and satisfied at meals. Research has shown that the body uses protein best when you space your intake throughout the day, rather than eating a large amount just once a day.

Protein comes from animal products, including meat, poultry, eggs, dairy, fish, seafood, and protein powder. Vegan sources of protein include soy products (such as tofu, tempeh, and edamame), seitan, legumes (beans, nuts, peas, and lentils), and seeds—and again, some protein powders.

Recommendations for healthy protein choices:

♦ Choose fish and seafood over red meat.

♦ Remove the skin from poultry.

♦ Choose lean or low-fat cuts of red meat. Limit or avoid fatty luncheon meats like salami, bologna, and hot dogs.

FATS

Fats are important for maintaining cell membranes and facilitating vitamin absorption, as well as other functions. Eating fat at meals can also help promote feelings of fullness. There are four major kinds of fat: monounsaturated, polyunsaturated, saturated, and trans fats. Generally speaking, you should choose the unsaturated types, limit saturated fats, and avoid trans fats.

Unsaturated fats, which are found in the Mediterranean diet, may actually reduce the risk of cardiovascular disease and improve glucose metabolism. A diet high in saturated fat is linked to elevated LDL (bad) cholesterol levels. There is some conflicting research on whether or not saturated fat increases the risk of heart disease. At this time, though, most experts still recommend that saturated fat intake be limited.

Recommendations for healthy fat choices:

♦ Avoid trans fats, which are found in stick margarine and many processed snack foods. Read the ingredient list on food labels for processed snack foods.

♦ Limit your intake of saturated fats, which are found in full-fat dairy, butter, well-marbled meat, and chicken fat and skin.

♦ Choose monounsaturated and polyunsaturated fats, which are found in olive oil, canola oil, and other vegetable oils; nuts and nut butters; seeds; avocado; and olives.

◆ Include omega-3 fats (a type of polyunsaturated fat) in your diet. They have numerous health benefits and are found in fatty fish such as salmon, trout, sardines, anchovies, and herring. Plant forms of omega-3 fats are found in flaxseeds, chia seeds, walnuts, canola oil, and leafy greens.

CARBOHYDRATES

Carbohydrates are your body's main source of energy. They are found in almost all foods, including the following:

Fruits

Fruits provide fiber, vitamins, minerals, and other nutrients that promote good health. Fruits contain more carbohydrates than most vegetables, so be careful with portion sizes.

Recommendations for healthy fruit choices:
◆ Choose fresh fruit over dried fruit and juice.
◆ If you buy frozen or canned fruit, choose those without added sugar.

Nonstarchy Vegetables

Think leafy greens, broccoli, cauliflower, peppers, asparagus, artichokes, tomatoes, and eggplant. These nonstarchy vegetables are low in calories and high in fiber, vitamins, minerals, and other nutrients that promote good health. They contain only a third as many carbohydrates as fruits, dairy, grains, beans, and starchy vegetables.

Recommendations for healthy vegetable choices:
◆ Choose a variety of vegetables, of all colors of the rainbow, to obtain a variety of nutrients.
◆ Buy fresh vegetables or frozen (with no added sauce). If you buy canned, look for low-sodium.
◆ Buy 100 percent vegetable juice, with no added fruit juice or sweeteners.

Grains, Beans, and Starchy Vegetables

Refined grains, such as white rice and white bread, have been processed to remove the bran, germ, and endosperm. They contain fewer nutrients and less fiber than whole grains. Beans and lentils are high in fiber and protein, as well as carbohydrate. Certain vegetables, such as corn, peas, and winter squash, are considered starchy because they contain more carbohydrates than nonstarchy vegetables. These vegetables are good sources of vitamins, minerals, fiber, and other nutrients that are important for good health.

Recommendations for healthy choices:

♦ At least half of all the grains you eat should be whole, not refined. Examples of whole-grain foods include whole-wheat bread, brown rice, quinoa, farro, millet, bulgur, wild rice, oatmeal, wheat berries, and barley.

♦ Include beans in your diet. Soak and cook them yourself, or buy them canned, drain out the liquid, and rinse.

♦ Buy starchy fresh vegetables or frozen (with no added sauce). If you buy canned, look for low-sodium.

Dairy

These are milk-based products and include milk, cheese, yogurt, and cottage cheese. Dairy products contain many nutrients, including calcium, protein, potassium, and vitamin D. Ideally, look for a brand that is fortified with calcium and vitamin D. Almond milk, cashew milk, soy milk, and hemp milk can all be good nondairy milk substitutes, as can leafy greens and tofu processed with calcium. All of these choices are very low in carbohydrates.

Recommendations for healthy dairy choices:

♦ Choose nonfat or low-fat dairy products or nondairy milk substitutes that are fortified with calcium and vitamin D.

♦ If you do choose full-fat dairy, keep portions moderate.

♦ Plain Greek yogurt, with 0 percent or 2 percent fat, contains half the amount of carbohydrate and double the protein of regular milk and yogurt.

FIBER

Fiber is the indigestible part of plants. It's found in vegetables, fruit, whole grains, legumes, and nuts. Despite the fact that most of it doesn't get digested, fiber does a lot of good things in the body. It contributes to digestive health and helps keep you feeling full longer. The soluble fiber (it absorbs water to form a gel) found in foods such as beans, lentils, and nonstarchy vegetables helps lower cholesterol and regulate blood sugar.

Recommendations to increase your fiber intake:

♦ Eat plenty of vegetables every day.

♦ Eat several servings of fruit a day.

♦ Choose whole grains over refined grains.

♦ Include beans and lentils in your diet.

SODIUM

Sodium is a mineral that helps maintain your electrolyte balance, as well as performing other functions in the body. However, excessive amounts may increase the risk for developing serious medical conditions such as high blood pressure, heart disease, and stroke. Since cardiovascular disease is the number one cause of illness and death in people with diabetes, it is especially important to limit your sodium intake. The majority of people's sodium intake comes from processed foods and restaurant meals—not the salt shaker.

People with diabetes should limit their sodium consumption to 2,300 milligrams (mg) a day. Lowering your sodium intake even more, to 1,500 mg a day, may benefit blood pressure in certain circumstances. The American Heart Association recommends 1,500 mg a day for African Americans; people diagnosed with hypertension, diabetes, or chronic kidney disease; and people over 51 years of age.

Recommendations to decrease sodium intake:

- Buy fresh or frozen (no sauce added) vegetables.
- Eat fresh poultry, fish, pork, and lean meat, rather than canned or processed meats.
- Buy low-sodium, lower sodium, reduced sodium, or no-salt-added versions of packaged products.
- Limit your use of sauces, mixes, and "instant products," including flavored rice and ready-made pasta.
- Read the Nutrition Facts labels on food packages for milligrams of sodium, and compare products.
- Review the sodium content of foods online before eating at chain restaurants.
- Limit using the salt shaker. (In the next chapter we give you alternative ways to season your food!)

Counting Carbs

How much carbohydrate should I eat a day? This is the number one question most people with diabetes ask. There is no one answer that's right for everyone. What is more important than the amount of carbohydrates per day is how they are distributed throughout the day in meals and snacks, to keep your blood sugar within a target range. Other factors to take into consideration when calculating goals for carbohydrate intake include your weight, age, activity level, food preferences, what medications you are taking, as well as any other medical issues.

Having diabetes does not mean you are doomed to follow a very low-carbohydrate diet. Your health-care team can give you more detailed guidance about the amount of carbohydrates you should eat each day. But in the meantime, here are two methods to help get you started: the plate method and carbohydrate counting.

BASIC: PLATE METHOD

The plate method is the simplest way to plan a diabetes-friendly meal. Most of my patients with newly diagnosed diabetes prefer to start with this method. It's an effective technique to ensure that your meals are balanced to achieve the right amount of carbs. Your plate should have the following ratios:

Protein: ¼ plate

Starch or grain: ¼ plate

Vegetables: ½ plate

Here are some tips to get you started with the plate method.

1 Use a nine-inch dinner plate. Portion control is easier when you have a smaller plate.

2 Imagine drawing a line down the middle of the plate. Divide one section in half again, so you have three sections on your plate.

3 Fill the largest section with nonstarchy vegetables such as green beans, Brussels sprouts, broccoli, cabbage, mushroom, zucchini, and salad greens. Any vegetable with fewer than 5 grams of carbohydrate per serving is considered nonstarchy. Refer to page 212–214 for a longer list of nonstarchy vegetables.

4 In one of the small sections, put grains and starchy foods such as rice, pasta, beans, potato, corn, peas, and bread.

5 In the other small section, put your protein, which might be fish, meat, poultry, eggs, tofu, cheese, nuts, or seeds.

6 In a small dessert cup, add one serving of fruit (one small fruit or ½ cup) or a serving of dairy (8 ounces nonfat or lowfat milk or yogurt)—or both, as your meal plan allows.

7 Choose healthy fats in moderation. Examples include cooking oils, vinaigrette salad dressing, nuts, seeds, and avocado.

8 Add a low-calorie drink such as water, seltzer, unsweetened tea, or coffee.

ADVANCED: CARBOHYDRATE COUNTING

One you have mastered the plate method, you may want to try carbohydrate counting as another way to plan meals. This method is quite flexible and lets you count grams of carbohydrates in your meals and snacks. Until you get more detailed guidance from your health-care team, here is a simple starting point for how many carbohydrates to eat in a day.

To lose weight

Women: 45 grams per meal and 15 grams for a snack

Men: 45 to 60 grams per meal and 15 to 30 grams for a snack

For weight maintenance

Women: 45 to 60 grams per meal and 15 to 30 grams for a snack

Men: 60 to 75 grams per meal and 30 grams for a snack

The American Diabetes Association recommends that people with diabetes eat no fewer than 130 grams of carbohydrate a day. However, some people find eating even fewer carbohydrates than this promotes better blood sugar control, and also helps weight management. If you would like to follow a lower carbohydrate diet, talk to your doctor and dietitian about a plan that is right for you.

To use this carb counting method, you will need to be familiar with where carbohydrates are found. As you have already learned, carbohydrates are found in many foods including grains, beans, fruit, dairy, many snack foods, and of course, sugar. To keep things simple, the various foods are grouped together here in portions that contain about the same amount of carbohydrate. Protein and fat contain no carbohydrates, as long as breading and sauces weren't used in their preparation. (You'll find a more detailed list of the carbohydrate content of foods on pages 213–214.)

Grains, starchy vegetables, and legumes

Each serving contains 15 grams of carbohydrate

- 1 slice (1 ounce) bread
- 2 slices light/diet bread
- ⅓ cup cooked rice, pasta, or quinoa
- ½ cup cooked hot cereal
- ¾ cup cold cereal (not a sugary brand)
- ½ cup sweet or mashed potato
- ½ medium potato (3 ounces)
- 1 (6-inch) corn or flour tortilla
- ½ cup plantain
- 1 cup winter squash
- 1 small ear of corn
- ½ cup beans or lentils
- ½ cup peas

Milk and yogurt

Each serving contains 12 grams of carbohydrate

+ 8 ounces milk

+ 8 ounces plain yogurt

+ 6 ounces artificially sweetened yogurt (read the labels on yogurt containers, because carbohydrate grams can vary widely)

Fruit

Each serving contains 15 grams of carbohydrate

+ 1 small apple, orange, peach, or nectarine

+ ½ grapefruit

+ ½ medium banana

+ 12 grapes or cherries

+ ½ cup canned unsweetened fruit or frozen fruit

Counting Carbs for a 1,500-Calorie Meal Plan

MEAL	TOTAL CARBS	FOOD CHOICES*
Breakfast	45 grams	2 slices whole-grain toast (30 grams) 1 teaspoon fat spread (0 grams) 1 egg (0 grams) ⅓ melon (15 grams)
Lunch	45 grams	4 ounces grilled chicken (0 grams) 2 cups greens (10 grams) 1 cup assorted raw vegetables (5 grams) 1 cup lentil soup (30 grams) 2 tablespoons vinaigrette dressing (0 grams)
Snack	15 grams	1 small apple (15 grams) 1 tablespoon almond butter (0 grams)

Dinner	40 grams	4 ounces broiled salmon (0 grams)
		⅔ cup brown rice (30 grams) with 1 teaspoon
		    fat spread (0 grams)
		1 cup steamed vegetables—broccoli, snow peas,
		    carrots (10 grams) cooked in 1 teaspoon oil (0 grams)

*The carbohydrate grams are averages.

Sweeteners

Each serving contains 15 grams of carbohydrate

♦ 1 tablespoon jam, jelly, honey, sugar, maple syrup, or agave

Nonstarchy vegetables

Each serving contains about 5 grams of carbohydrate

♦ ½ cup cooked

♦ 1 cup raw

Carbohydrate-containing snack foods

Each serving contains 15 grams of carbohydrate

♦ ¾ ounce crackers

♦ ¾ ounce pretzels

♦ 3 cups air-popped popcorn

♦ 3 cups low-fat microwave popcorn

♦ 10 to 12 baked potato chips

The carbohydrate content of snack food varies widely, so your best bet is to read the label for portion size and grams of carbohydrate. You can find many snack ideas for 15 and 30 grams of carbohydrate on pages 78 and 79.

Combination foods

Foods such as soup, pizza, casseroles, and other mixed dishes usually contain a combination of protein, fat, and carbohydrates. The exact amount of carbohydrate depends on the portion size and how the dish is made. You will find the carbohydrate content of the recipes in this book listed with the recipe. For other items, such as soup or pizza, you can check the food label for the carbohydrate content or use a calorie and carbohydrate counting app such as CalorieKing.com.

I'm sure you will come across a food that doesn't fit into the lists here. This is where carbohydrate counting can be very flexible. If you are dining out, refer to the restaurant's website. For example, the Subway website states that a six-inch turkey sandwich on whole-wheat bread with lettuce, peppers, tomato, cucumber, and mustard has 330 calories and 46 grams of carbs. Add a water and you have a diabetes-friendly meal on the go. You can also check out websites like CalorieKing.com to see the carbohydrate content of your favorite foods. And of course, read the labels of your favorite foods for the exact carbohydrate content.

Carbs and Calories of Common Foods

You may be surprised to see the large amounts of carbohydrates (and calories!) in your favorite foods and beverages.

Starbucks Grande Iced Chai Latte: 44 grams carbs, 240 calories

Starbucks Grande Caffè Mocha with 2 percent milk: 42 grams carbs, 290 calories

Dunkin Donuts Everything Bagel: 67 grams carbs, 340 calories

Vitamin Water Acai-Blueberry-Pomegranate (20-ounce bottle): 31 grams carbs, 120 calories

Jamba Juice Banana Berry Smoothie, medium: 92 grams carbs, 390 calories

Pizzeria Uno Individual Size Deep Dish Pizza (cheese and tomato): 117 grams carbs, 1,750 calories

Chipotle Chicken Burrito (tortilla, rice, pinto beans, cheese, chicken, sour cream, guacamole, salsa): 122 grams carbs, 1,275 calories (plus 60 grams fat, 2,790 mg sodium)

PF Chang's Cantonese-Style Lemon Chicken with White Rice: 182 grams carbs, 1,410 calories (plus 43 grams fat, 1,511 mg sodium)

Applebee's American Standard Burger with Classic Fries: 107 grams carbs, 1,469 calories (plus 91 grams fat, 2,740 mg sodium)

How to Read a Label

Reading food labels is an important tool to help you figure out what you are eating. Food labels contain a lot of information, but here is what I consider the most important:

Serving size: Pay close attention, as most of us eat more than one serving.

Calories: Helpful for weight control.

Total Carbohydrates: Very useful if you are counting grams of carbohydrates. Focus on Total Carbohydrates rather than Sugar. All carbohydrates turn into sugar in your blood. So even if a product claims to be sugar-free and has 0 grams of sugar, if it contains 40 grams of carbohydrate, eating this food will still raise your blood sugar.

Fiber: Helps slow the rise of blood sugar, helps lower cholesterol, and keeps you feeling full for longer.

Sugar: While it is recommended that you keep your sugar intake to a minimum, sugar on the label does not distinguish between sugar found naturally in nutrient-rich foods like fruit and milk, and added sugars found in soda, candy, and desserts.

Sodium, protein, and saturated fat are also important. So is the ingredients list. This is where you will find exactly what is in the food. Look for whole grains (which you want!), and try to limit added sugars such as agave and high-fructose corn syrup, hydrogenated oils, and saturated and trans fats.

Stay tuned for the new food labels that will roll out in 2017 and be mandatory by 2019. There will be many changes, but here are the most important ones:

♦ Larger serving sizes that are more consistent with the way Americans eat.

♦ Calories will be more prominently listed.

♦ A new category of Added Sugars under Total Sugars, along with daily recommendations; this will help distinguish between the sugars found naturally in foods and the hidden added sugar in foods like soda, cereal, and granola bars.

Nutrition Facts

Serving Size 2/3 cup (55g)
Servings Per Container About 8

Amount Per Serving

Calories 230	Calories from Fat 72

	% Daily Value*
Total Fat 8g	**12%**
Saturated Fat 1g	**5%**
Trans Fat 0g	
Cholesterol 0mg	**0%**
Sodium 160mg	**7%**
Total Carbohydrate 37g	**12%**
Dietary Fiber 4g	**16%**
Sugars 1g	
Protein 3g	

Vitamin A	10%
Vitamin C	8%
Calcium	20%
Iron	45%

* Percent Daily Values are based on a 2,000 calorie diet. Your daily value may be higher or lower depending on your calorie needs.

	Calories:	2,000	2,500
Total Fat	Less than	65g	80g
Sat Fat	Less than	20g	25g
Cholesterol	Less than	300mg	300mg
Sodium	Less than	2,400mg	2,400mg
Total Carbohydrate		300g	375g
Dietary Fiber		25g	30g

Nutrition Facts

8 servings per container
Serving size   2/3 cup (55g)

Amount per serving
Calories   230

	% Daily Value*
Total Fat 8g	**10%**
Saturated Fat 1g	**5%**
Trans Fat 0g	
Cholesterol 0mg	**0%**
Sodium 160mg	**7%**
Total Carbohydrate 37g	**13%**
Dietary Fiber 4g	**14%**
Total Sugars 12g	
Includes 10g Added Sugars	**20%**
Protein 3g	

Vitamin D 2mcg	10%
Calcium 260mg	20%
Iron 8mg	45%
Potassium 235mg	6%

* The % Daily Value (DV) tells you how much a nutrient in a serving of food contributes to a daily diet. 2,000 calories a day is used for general nutrition advice.

http://www.fda.gov/Food/GuidanceRegulation/GuidanceDocumentsRegulatoryInformation/LabelingNutrition/ucm385663.htm

All Carbs Are Not Created Equal

As we've already mentioned, all carbohydrates raise blood sugar and therefore should be eaten in moderation. For those of you who are counting carbs, you know that one slice of bread has 15 grams of carbohydrate, whether it is white bread or whole-wheat bread. So you may wonder why whole-wheat bread is the better choice, since they contain the same amount of carbohydrates. Good question!

To start with, whole-wheat bread has more nutrients. But there is another reason, too: All carbs are not created equal. Different foods containing carbohydrates affect blood sugar levels differently. These effects can be quantified by measures known as the glycemic index and the glycemic load.

GLYCEMIC INDEX

The glycemic index (GI) tells you how quickly a particular carbohydrate in a food causes blood sugar to rise. Foods are ranked on a scale of 0 to 100, with pure sugar given a value of 100. The lower a food's glycemic index, the slower blood sugar rises after eating that food; the higher the number, the more rapid the rise.

While many studies show GI is a useful tool in managing blood sugar, not all experts agree. First of all, the GI is based on eating the food alone. How many times do you have a slice of white bread all by itself? Most of us would add butter and/or an egg. Adding protein, fat, and fiber to a meal lowers the GI. And in general, the more processed or cooked a food is, the higher the GI.

I find that the GI can be a helpful tool . . . but don't read into it too strictly. For example, peanut M&Ms have a GI of 33, as compared to an orange, which has a GI of 45—and we know the orange is a healthier choice!

GLYCEMIC LOAD

Many experts believe that the glycemic load (GL) is a better tool than the GI. Like the GI, it assesses the impact of a food on blood sugar. But it gives a more comprehensive picture because it takes into account how much carbohydrate is available in a serving of food. Here is an example: Watermelon has a high glycemic index of 72, but also has a high percentage of water, so the GL is only 4.

Bottom line, the total amount of carbohydrates you eat and how you space them out is what is most important. The type of carbohydrates can play a role as well. Foods with a lower GL, such as vegetables, whole grains, fruit, and plain yogurt, tend to be less processed and healthier overall compared to foods with a higher GL. So select foods as close to their natural state as often as possible.

Food affects each individual's blood sugar differently. For those of you testing your blood sugar after meals, pay attention to how various foods affect your blood sugar. Chances are the lower GL foods will have less of an impact. (See pages 209–212 for a detailed list of the GI and GL of common foods.)

Swaps for lowering GI and GL:

+ Instead of white rice, choose quinoa, brown rice, or barley.

+ Instead of instant oatmeal, choose steel-cut oats.

+ Instead of a baked potato, choose a yam or lentils.

+ Instead of raisins, choose an apple.

+ Instead of white bread, choose whole-grain bread.

How Many Calories Should You Eat per Day?

In the next chapter, you will find meal plans for 1,500, 1,800, and 2,100 calories per day. It is helpful to understand how many calories your body needs each day. Your caloric need depends on several factors, including weight, height, age, activity level, body composition, and whether you want to lose, maintain, or gain weight.

Since 80 percent of people with type 2 diabetes are overweight, I find that the majority of my patients are interested in losing weight. It can be difficult to predict exactly how many calories your body needs to accomplish this, due to variations in individual metabolism. An average woman needs about 1,700 to 2,000 calories per day to maintain her weight and 1,200 to 1,500 calories to lose one pound a week. An average man needs 1,800 to 2,300 calories to maintain, and 1,500 to 1,800 to lose one pound a week. Health experts generally recommend that most people who want to lose weight should aim to lose one to two pounds a week.

Here are two quick formulas to calculate your caloric needs:

FOR WEIGHT MAINTENANCE

+ 10 calories per pound if you are overweight, sedentary (a lifestyle with little or no activity), and have a difficult time losing weight.

+ 13 calories per pound if you are overweight and moderately active (engaging in physical activity equivalent to walking about 1.5 to 3 miles per day at 3 to 4 miles per hour).

+ 15 calories—or more—per pound if you are active (engaging in physical activity equivalent to walking more than 3 miles per day at 3 to 4 miles per hour).

FOR WEIGHT LOSS

◆ To lose 1 pound a week, subtract 500 calories from your maintenance calorie level.

◆ To lose 2 pounds a week, subtract 1,000 calories from your maintenance calorie level.

For a more accurate way to calculate caloric needs, try an online calorie calculator. You'll find them at USDA Caloric Needs Calculator (fnic.nal.usda.gov) and CalorieKing.com. Here is some food for thought when it comes to calories: Just as not all carbohydrates are created equal, neither are calories. Studies have shown that it's more efficient for the body to break down highly processed foods compared to foods that are higher in fiber and protein. Your body has to work harder to digest these protein- and fiber-rich foods and actually burns calories doing so. So 100 calories from healthy food such as almonds, broccoli, or salmon aren't the same as 100 calories from cookies, white bread, or potato chips. In addition, newer research is suggesting that the best strategy is to consume the majority of your calories from foods that are as unprocessed as possible.

Healthy Meal Planning for Diabetes

We've reviewed the major nutrients, calories, carbohydrate counting, and food labels. Now it's time to put it all together. A diabetic diet is not just about limiting carbohydrates. A healthy, diabetes-friendly diet will help you control your blood sugar, decrease the risk of complications, and promote weight loss if you are overweight.

Of course, you can occasionally fit in your favorite candy bar, but that should be a rare treat! What is more important is what you eat every day. I know it can be difficult to make changes in your eating habits, so you may want to start with just a few of these suggestions, and add more as you feel comfortable with the changes.

1 Try to eat meals on a regular schedule. Not only does this help stabilize blood sugar, but it can also help keep energy levels up and prevent you overeating at your next meal.

2 Control the portions of all carbohydrate-containing foods, especially grains, starchy vegetables, beans, fruit, milk, most processed snack foods, and of course, sweeteners. All carbohydrates will raise blood sugar.

3 Eat balanced meals that include carbohydrate, protein, and fat. The protein helps you feel fuller longer and the fat helps stabilize blood sugar longer. For example, a slice of toast alone would likely cause a more rapid rise of blood sugar than a slice of toast with 2 teaspoons of natural peanut butter. Preventing spikes of blood sugar can also help your pancreas, because it will not have to produce large amounts of insulin to lower the blood sugar. This can help lessen insulin resistance.

4 Fiber is your friend. Not only does it aid in gastrointestinal health, but it may also help lower cholesterol and prevent blood sugar spikes after a meal.

5 Keep highly processed foods to a minimum. The more processed a food is, the fewer nutrients it contains, and often times, the quicker the rise in blood sugar.

6 Fill up on nonstarchy vegetables. They are loaded with nutrients and high in fiber, and they also have a minimal effect on raising blood sugar and will keep you feeling full without the calories.

7 Use the glycemic index and glycemic load as guides to fine-tune your carbohydrate choices.

8 Make it easy for yourself. Keep healthy foods in the house. Buy smaller plates and bowls. Research ahead of time what you can eat at your local restaurants. (We'll talk more about this in the next chapter.)

9 All calories count if you are trying to lose weight. (We'll discuss more about portion sizes and tracking your calories in the next chapter.)

10 And best of all, try out our delicious recipes. We've done all the work for you by calculating the calories and carbohydrates.

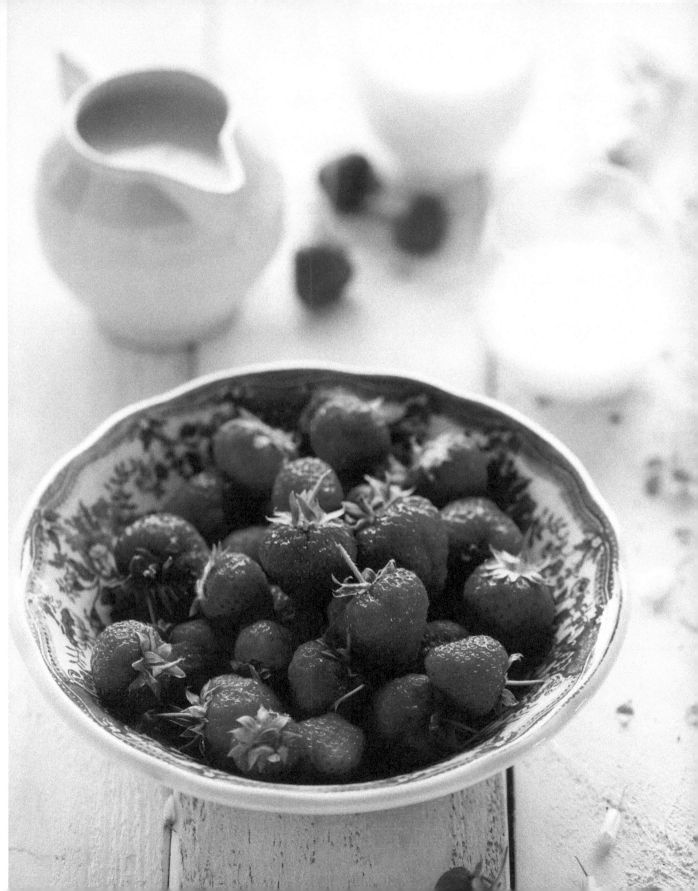

CHAPTER 2

Plan Your Health, Work Your Plan

It's not easy to make changes in your eating habits. While it can take years to develop new habits, we are going to guide you on how you can start to make changes toward healthful eating habits. We want to keep it as simple as possible for you and will spell everything out for the first month.

The first goal will be to stock your kitchen with healthy ingredients, and purge the not-so-healthy ones. Then get ready to make the delicious diabetes-friendly recipes in this book. There are plenty of make-ahead meals and meals that use leftovers to make the adjustment as easy as possible. You'll find that it's simple to make meals that the whole family enjoys, and that help you control your blood sugar and watch your weight.

Stocking Your Kitchen

Having a kitchen stocked with healthy foods is key to helping you make smart choices every day and maintain long-term healthy eating habits. Remember that foods that are healthy for people with diabetes also have great benefits for those without diabetes. When you're grocery shopping, read food labels and stick to foods that are processed as little as possible, to increase nutritional value and lower the glycemic index.

Purge your kitchen of tempting not-so-healthy foods, including sweets like cookies, soda, ice cream, and high-sugar cereals and snacks. If it's not there, you can't eat it!

The recipes in this book should seem familiar to most of you. The ingredients are common, easy to find, and full of flavor. In some cases, we suggest ways you can add to or change the recipes. Please remember that if you make any changes, the nutrient profile will change too.

In this chapter we also give you ideas for some extra flavor boosters, and some essential equipment. If you're feeling a bit overwhelmed right now, start by making small changes. Try to add in a few healthy foods each week.

THE PANTRY

Canned tomatoes and tomato sauce (low-sodium)

Canned tuna and salmon, packed in water

Chia seeds

Ground flaxseed

Healthy vegetable oils, including extra-virgin olive oil and canola oil

Low-sodium canned and dried broth

Low-sodium canned bean soups

Low-sodium dried or canned beans and lentils

Low-sugar jam and jelly

Nonstick cooking spray

Nut butters like natural peanut butter and almond butter (low-sodium)

Steel-cut oatmeal

Sweet potatoes

Tomato paste

Unsalted nuts

Vinegar

Whole-grain bread (look for at least 2 grams of fiber per slice)

Whole-grain cereal (look for at least 5 grams of fiber per serving)

Whole-grain crackers (look for at least 2 grams of fiber per serving)

Whole-grain sides such as brown rice, whole-wheat pasta, quinoa, barley, buckwheat, and farro

Whole-wheat tortillas

THE FREEZER

Edamame

Frozen fruit

Frozen vegetables without sauce

Lean protein like chicken, turkey, lean beef, lean cuts of pork (such as tenderloin)

Frozen meals as a backup (less than 500 mg of sodium, at least 15 grams of protein, 45 grams of carbohydrates or less, at least 6 grams of fiber, 400 calories or less)

THE REFRIGERATOR

A variety of fresh fruit

A variety of nonstarchy vegetables

Cheese (preferably low-fat), including grated Parmesan cheese, single-serving sizes like string cheese and Babybel

Dijon mustard

Eggs

Low-calorie beverages like seltzer

Low-sodium vegetable juice

Nonfat and lowfat milk

Nonfat and lowfat yogurt (preferably plain Greek)

Nondairy milk alternatives (almond milk, coconut milk, and soy milk)

Vegan sources of protein like tofu, tempeh, and seitan

FLAVOR BOOSTERS

Here are ways to add flavor without the sugar, sodium, and calories found in most other flavor enhancers. These are essential for a diabetes-friendly kitchen.

Flavored vinegars such as pomegranate, raspberry, and fig

Fresh or dried herbs and spices, including allspice, basil, black pepper, cayenne pepper, cinnamon, cumin, oregano, red pepper flakes, and rosemary

Garlic and onions

Ginger, freshly grated and ground

Hot sauce

Lemon and lime, juice and zest

Low-sodium soy sauce

No-salt seasonings such as Mrs. Dash

Salsa

Sriracha sauce

ESSENTIAL EQUIPMENT

In addition to the basic pots and pans, you'll need some tools for weighing and measuring. For some foods, that's the most accurate way to calculate calories and grams of carbohydrates. Here are a few other pieces of equipment that are essential for a diabetes-friendly kitchen:

+ Blender or food processor
+ Kitchen scale
+ Measuring cups and spoons
+ Vegetable spiralizer (spiralized zucchini is a great replacement for pasta—without the calories or carbohydrates)
+ Vegetable steamer

Fine-Tuning Your Eating Plan

In chapter 1 we talked about the basics of a healthy diet, including the nutrients your body needs for good health, carbohydrate and calorie counting, and reading food labels. Now we will get into a little more detail, talking about issues that people with type 2 diabetes frequently ask. Will having a glass of wine spike blood sugar? Should you use real sugar or an artificial one? How should you measure portion sizes? Here is where you learn how to fine-tune your eating plan.

PORTION CONTROL

Considering that 70 percent of Americans are overweight or obese, it's safe to say that most of our portions are too large. The best way to get an idea of what your portion sizes are is to weigh or measure them. Buy a food scale to weigh cheese, nuts, meat, fish, chicken, and potatoes. Get out your measuring cups to measure cold and hot cereal, cooked pasta, rice and other grains, and beverages. Use measuring spoons to measure salad dressings, oil, and peanut butter.

And if you don't have measuring cups or spoons handy, use these visuals:

+ 2 dice = 1 teaspoon
+ Your thumb from knuckle to tip = 1 tablespoon
+ Golf ball or wine cork = 2 tablespoons
+ Matchbox or Tic-Tac container = 1 ounce meat or cheese
+ Deck of cards = 3 ounces
+ Computer mouse or ½ baseball = ½ cup
+ Baseball or tennis ball = 1 cup

WATCH WHAT YOU EAT

Most of us vastly underestimate what we eat. We tend to graze during the day and forget what we have eaten. Or we aren't aware of our portion sizes.

Studies have shown that keeping a food log can increase your weight loss by 50 percent! Even if you aren't trying to lose weight, a food log can make you more aware of your carbohydrate intake, which will help with blood sugar management. Record the time you eat or drink, as well as the portion size. Try to write it down as soon after eating as possible. To get an accurate sense of your portion size, it is best to weigh and/or measure some food and beverages. If you don't have the measuring tools handy, use the visuals we've provided as a guide.

It can also be helpful to log your degree of hunger or any emotions you are feeling, and use the information to make observations and adjustments. Are you craving sugar in the afternoon because you didn't have any protein at lunch? Is your diet lacking in fruits and vegetables? Do you tend to eat for emotional reasons?

You can keep your food log in a notebook or on an app. Some popular apps include MyFitnessPal, MyNetDiary, Livestrong, and Lose It.

ALCOHOL

My patients frequently ask me about alcohol. The good news is that alcohol can easily fit into a healthy diabetes diet. Contrary to popular belief, alcohol has minimal impact on raising blood sugar. In fact, it may cause low blood sugar if you are taking insulin or certain diabetes medications, and if alcohol is consumed without food.

Dry wine or hard liquor with low-sugar mixers are the best choices and contain negligible amounts of carbohydrates. Sweet wine and beer tend to contain more carbohydrates, so if you do drink those, be sure to include the carbohydrates into your meal plan. Avoid or limit those drinks made with sweet mixers such as rum and coke or Piña Coladas. You can refer to websites such as CalorieKing.com for the calories and carbohydrates of alcoholic drinks.

All alcohol should be consumed in moderation, whether you have diabetes or not, for your overall health. Women should have no more than one drink a day. Men should have no more than two drinks a day. One drink is equal to 12 ounces of beer, 5 ounces of wine, or 1½ ounces of distilled spirits (vodka, whiskey, gin, etc.).

SUGAR SUBSTITUTES

The average American consumes 22 teaspoons of sugar a day, for a whopping 355 calories. People with diabetes often ask me if sugar substitutes are a better choice than real sugar. Sugar substitutes, also known as nonnutritive sweeteners or artificial sweeteners, contain few or no carbohydrates and calories and have minimal effect on blood sugar. Examples include aspartame, acesulfame-K, Neotame, saccharin, and sucralose. Another sugar substitute is stevia, which comes from a plant.

On-the-Fly Meals

These quick meals come together in just a few minutes, using ingredients you likely have on hand. (The calorie and carbohydrate numbers here are estimates.)

EGG SCRAMBLE 1

1 egg, vegetables (chopped tomatoes, peppers, mushrooms, or whatever you have around), cooked using nonstick cooking spray

1 slice whole-grain toast, spread with 1 teaspoon healthy fat
(butter or nonhydrogenated spread)

½ grapefruit or any other fruit

Method: Scramble egg with vegetables, serve with buttered toast and grapefruit.

290 calories, 30 grams carbohydrates

EGG SCRAMBLE 2

2 eggs, vegetables (chopped tomatoes, peppers, mushrooms, or whatever you have around), cooked using nonstick cooking spray

2 slices whole-grain toast, spread with 1 teaspoon healthy fat
(butter or nonhydrogenated spread)

½ grapefruit or any other fruit

Method: Scramble eggs with vegetables, serve with buttered toast and grapefruit.

450 calories, 45 grams carbohydrates

YOGURT PARFAIT

6 ounces (¾ cup) 0 percent or 2 percent plain Greek yogurt

¾ cup mixed berries

1 tablespoon pumpkin seeds

Method: Top yogurt with berries and seeds.

225 calories, 23 grams carbohydrates

QUICK TACOS

1 medium whole-wheat tortilla (1.6 ounces)

½ cup kidney, black, or pinto beans

1.5 ounces or ⅓ cup low-fat shredded cheese

4 tablespoons salsa

2 tablespoons light sour cream

Method: Place beans and cheese on the tortilla and microwave until warm, about 90 seconds. Top with salsa and sour cream.

420 calories, 50 grams carbohydrates

TUNA PASTA SALAD

2 ounces whole-wheat pasta, cooked

1 tablespoon extra-virgin olive oil

1 tablespoon wine vinegar

3 ounces canned tuna, packed in water (drained)

1 cup assorted vegetables

Method: In a large bowl, toss all ingredients together, then serve.

435 calories, 50 grams carbohydrates

TURKEY SANDWICH

2 slices whole-grain bread

4 ounces cooked turkey breast

¼ avocado, sliced

Dijon mustard

2 leaves lettuce

½ tomato, sliced

Method: Spread mustard on one slice of bread. Top with turkey, avocado, lettuce, tomato, and remaining slice of bread.

380 calories, 30 grams carbohydrates

PROTEIN-PACKED SALMON SALAD

4 ounces leftover cooked salmon

2 to 3 cups mixed greens tossed with an assortment of nonstarchy vegetables (tomatoes, carrots, cucumbers, leftover cooked vegetables)

½ cup cooked chickpeas, rinsed and drained if canned

5 olives

2 tablespoons low-fat vinaigrette

1 small whole-grain roll (1 ounce)

Method: In a large bowl, combine salmon, mixed greens and vegetables, chickpeas, and olives. Top with vinaigrette and serve with roll.

510 calories, 45 grams carbohydrates

Sugar substitutes are found in many foods and beverages, including diet soda and other dietetic products. Compare a 12-ounce diet soda, which has 0 calories and 0 grams of carbohydrate, to a regular soda with 155 calories and 40 grams of carbohydrate.

People have debated the safety of artificial sweeteners for years. The FDA has approved them as safe, and people with diabetes and those trying to lose weight have used them for years. The FDA also considers stevia as generally recognized as safe (GRAS).

To date, researchers have found no clear evidence that these sweeteners cause cancer or other serious health problems in humans. However, some research suggests that artificial sweeteners can affect the microbes in our gut that digest food, which in turn can impair some people's ability to process glucose. Other studies suggest the intensely sweet taste of artificial sweeteners may lead to a preference for sweet foods, which may lead to overeating. It is also possible that artificial sweeteners lead to an increased intake of calories later in the day, beyond what would have been consumed in the absence of the use of these sweeteners. But more studies need to be done to conclusively prove any of these possibilities.

The decision is yours. Your best bet is to choose moderation—whether it be a real sugar or a nonnutritive sweetener. If you do choose a real sugar, just keep in mind that 1 tablespoon contains 15 grams of carbohydrate. If you are testing your own blood sugar, pay attention to how sugar affects you.

SUGAR ALCOHOLS

Sugar alcohols are neither sugar nor alcohol. They are simple carbohydrates that have been chemically modified to provide a sweet taste with half the carbohydrates of other sugars. Unlike artificial sweeteners, sugar alcohols can raise blood sugar levels because they are carbohydrates. But because your body does not completely absorb sugar alcohols, their effect on blood sugar is less than that of other sugars.

You will find them in sugar-free and reduced-sugar versions of candies, cookies, baked goods, syrups, and frozen desserts. Examples include sorbitol, mannitol, erythritol, and maltitol. If it ends in "ol," it is likely a sugar alcohol. Because they are incompletely digested, you can subtract half of the sugar alcohol grams from the total carbohydrate count, if you are counting grams of carbohydrate in your meal plan. But beware, because eating foods with a lot of sugar alcohols may cause gas or have a laxative effect.

Move It

What is one thing you can do that has a positive effect on almost every part of your body—brain, heart, muscles, bones, blood pressure, and even blood sugar? Exercise! Regular physical activity is a key part of managing diabetes—along with proper meal planning and, if needed, medication.

Exercise helps lower blood glucose by increasing the muscles' ability to take up and use blood glucose. It can also lower the amount of medication needed to keep blood glucose levels in the target range. And if that were not enough, regular physical activity is important for your overall well-being; it can help with many other health conditions, including decreasing the risk of heart disease and stroke, improving circulation, and lowering blood pressure.

Unfortunately, most of us don't do enough of it! Only 20 percent of US adults are meeting both the aerobic and muscle-strengthening components of the federal government's physical activity recommendations, according to the Centers for Disease Control and Prevention. The physical activity guidelines, developed by the American College of Sports Medicine and the American Diabetes Association, recommend a minimum of 150 minutes a week of aerobic exercise at moderate intensity or greater and at least two sessions a week of resistance training exercise. Regular physical activity is an extremely important part of any diabetes treatment plan. In the next chapter, we will talk more about the benefits of regular exercise and give you tips to get started and stay active.

Whole Health

When you have diabetes, it is not unusual to feel overwhelmed by your eating and exercise plan and possibly having to take medications and check your blood sugar daily. Diabetes is a 24-hour-a-day, seven-day-a-week disease. Probably the last thing on your mind is the state of your mental health.

However, good emotional health is key to managing your diabetes for the long term. The daily stress of having diabetes can add up. Or you may feel frustrated or sad if you are having trouble controlling your blood sugar or are experiencing complications. People with diabetes also have a greater risk of depression than people without diabetes. This is a vicious cycle because feeling overwhelmed, stressed, or depressed can interfere with you taking care of your diabetes. You may not feel like eating healthily, exercising, or taking your medication.

I have had many patients tell me they feel frustrated and even angry when they are diagnosed and learn that they have to restrict certain foods and test their blood sugar. What has helped my clients is learning to take charge of their diabetes instead of it controlling them—specifically by learning how to manage stress, becoming more mindful, taking time out, and coming up with a plan to deal with social challenges. In the next chapter you will find tips on what you can do to keep yourself emotionally as well as physically healthy.

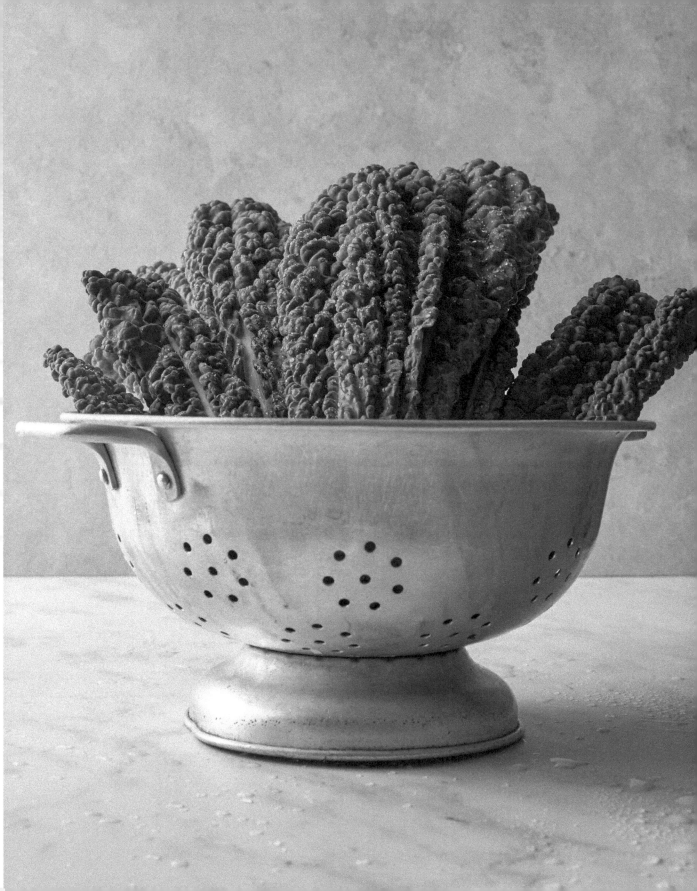

CHAPTER 3

The Plan

This chapter is all about healthy diabetes-friendly food and tasty meals for you and your family. Get ready to start cooking! We'll keep it simple and tell you exactly what to buy and how to prepare it. The goal for the first month is to get you used to cooking meals in a healthy way, with the right portion sizes to help keep your blood sugar in good control.

Then in the second month we add in some physical activity, which also plays a vital role in blood sugar management, weight control, and overall health. You'll get practical tips to get you moving, as well as suggestions on how to manage stress.

In the third month the focus is on mental and emotional well-being as it relates to diabetes. This area is often neglected but is an important part of diabetes self-management. We also discuss common diabetes-related challenges, and give you practical tips for dealing with social situations like restaurant dining, holidays, and parties.

Month One

Month one is all about the meal plans. Being diagnosed with diabetes can feel overwhelming, so we want to help you by taking all the guesswork out of what you can eat. You'll get specific meal plans for breakfast, lunch, dinner, and snacks for the next two weeks. If the name of a dish in the plan begins with capital letters—Like This—it means there is a recipe for it in this book.

After the first two weeks, you can just follow the same meal plan again. Or, since you will have a better sense of what to eat, you can use the recipes in this book to plan your diet for the rest of the month. Just make sure that the calories and carbohydrate grams in the recipes are similar to the ones in the meal plan. We know there may be some dishes you like better than others, so feel free to substitute another recipe for one listed here. Again, just be sure it has a very similar calorie and carb profile.

You'll see that there are two snacks included every day. While we have placed them midmorning and midafternoon, you can have them whenever you want. Some people like to have a snack after dinner, and that is perfectly fine.

We've even included shopping lists so you will know exactly what to buy at the supermarket. The shopping lists show what you will need for the week, making the recipes as they're written, to serve four people. Of course, when you buy staples like ground spices and honey, one jar will last awhile and you won't have to keep throwing them in your shopping cart week after week. The lists are based on the recipes we've included in the meal plans, so if you choose different recipes, you'll have to adjust your shopping list. And while we've suggested snacks in every meal plan, we've left them off the shopping lists, because we want you to have the flexibility to choose your own snacks.

You'll find three different calorie levels for the meal plans, since not all people have the same calorie and carbohydrate needs. To figure out which calorie level is right for you, check How Many Calories Should You Eat a Day? (page 28), for guidance. In general, most women trying to lose weight should aim for 1,500 calories a day, and 1,800 calories to maintain their weight. Most men should aim for 1,800 calories to lose weight and 2,100 calories to maintain their weight. Once you have picked your appropriate calorie level meal plans, you don't need to worry about the right amount of carbohydrates, as we have already figured that out for you. If you find you are still hungry, eat more nonstarchy vegetables.

Get ready to make some delicious meals!

1,500-CALORIE WEEKLY MEAL PLANS AND SHOPPING LISTS

WEEK 1 MEAL PLAN

MONDAY

Breakfast: Cottage Cheese Almond Pancakes with ½ cup raspberries

Snack: ½ medium apple, and 1 teaspoon almond butter

Lunch: Chicken and Roasted Vegetable Wrap

Snack: ¼ cup hummus, and 1 ounce whole-grain pretzels

Dinner: Spicy Citrus Sole, and Quinoa Vegetable Skillet (double the recipes so you'll have leftovers for tomorrow)

Total Carbs Per Day: 145g

TUESDAY

Breakfast: Fruity Avocado Smoothie

Snack: 10 to 12 almonds

Lunch: Leftover Spicy Citrus Sole, and Quinoa Vegetable Skillet

Snack: ½ cup low-fat cottage cheese, and 1 medium peach

Dinner: Lime-Parsley Lamb Cutlets, and Zucchini Noodles with Lime-Basil Pesto (double the recipes so you'll have leftovers for tomorrow)

Total Carbs Per Day: 135g

WEDNESDAY

Breakfast: Sweet Quinoa Cereal

Snack: ¼ cup pomegranate seeds, and 4 ounces 2 percent plain Greek yogurt

Lunch: Leftover Lime-Parsley Lamb Cutlets, and Zucchini Noodles with Lime-Basil Pesto

Snack: 2 ounces smoked salmon, tomato slices, 1 tablespoon low-fat cream cheese on 2 high-fiber crackers

Dinner: Pork Chop Diane, and Roasted Eggplant with Goat Cheese (double the recipes so you'll have leftovers for tomorrow)

Total Carbs Per Day: 139g

THURSDAY

Breakfast: 2 Lemon Blueberry Muffins with 1 teaspoon butter, and 1 cup sliced strawberries

Snack: ⅓ avocado, and 1 whole-wheat English muffin

Lunch: Leftover Pork Chop Diane, and Roasted Eggplant with Goat Cheese

Snack: 3 tablespoons hummus, and 1 cup assorted raw vegetables

Dinner: Tantalizing Jerked Chicken, and Mediterranean Chickpea Slaw (double the recipes so you'll have leftovers for tomorrow)

Total Carbs Per Day: 145g

FRIDAY

Breakfast: Wild Mushroom Frittata

Snack: 1 medium banana, and 1 tablespoon peanut butter

Lunch: Leftover Tantalizing Jerked Chicken, and Mediterranean Chickpea Slaw

Snack: ½ small whole-wheat pita (½-ounce), and ½ ounce low-fat cheese spread

Dinner: Mediterranean Steak Sandwich, and Pico de Gallo Navy Beans (double the recipes so you'll have leftovers for tomorrow)

Total Carbs Per Day: 144g

SATURDAY

Breakfast: Pumpkin Apple Waffles

Snack: ¼ cup shelled sunflower seeds

Lunch: Leftover Mediterranean Steak Sandwich, and Pico de Gallo Navy Beans

Snack: ½ cup Breyer's No Sugar Added Vanilla ice cream

Dinner: Haddock with Creamy Cucumber Sauce, and Fennel and Chickpeas (double the recipes so you'll have leftovers for tomorrow)

Total Carbs Per Day: 150g

SUNDAY

Breakfast: 2 Lemon Blueberry Muffins

Snack: 1 Enlightened ice cream bar

Lunch: Leftover Haddock with Creamy Cucumber Sauce, and Fennel and Chickpeas

Snack: 8 or 9 cashew halves

Dinner: Juicy Turkey Burger on a whole-wheat bun, and Sautéed Mixed Vegetables (double the recipes so you'll have leftovers for tomorrow)

Total Carbs Per Day: 150g

WEEK 1 SHOPPING LIST

MEAT AND SEAFOOD

chicken breasts, boneless, skinless
(2 [8 ounce] and 8 [5 ounce])

flank steak (2 pounds)

ground turkey (3 pounds)

haddock fillets (8 [5 ounce])

lamb cutlets (24 [about 3 pounds total])

pork top loin chops, boneless (8 [5 ounce])

sole fillets (8 [6 ounces each])

DAIRY, DAIRY ALTERNATIVES, AND EGGS

almond milk, unsweetened plain (2 cups)

butter (3 tablespoons)

cottage cheese, low-fat (2 cups)

eggs (22)

feta cheese, low-sodium (12 ounces)

goat cheese (¾ cup)

Greek yogurt, 2 percent, plain (1¼ cups)

milk, skim (2½ cups)

PRODUCE

apple (1)

avocado (1)

banana (1)

basil, fresh (4 bunches)

blueberries (1½ cups)

broccoli (2 heads)

carrots (6)

cauliflower (2 heads)

PRODUCE continued

chives, fresh (1 bunch)

corn kernels, fresh or frozen (2 cups)

eggplant (1)

English cucumbers (3)

fennel bulbs (2)

garlic (1 head)

green beans (2 cups)

habanero chile peppers (4)

jalapeño pepper (1)

kale (1 bunch)

lemons (2)

lettuce (1 head)

limes (12)

mint, fresh (1 bunch)

mushrooms, cremini, oyster, shiitake, portobello, etc. (2 cups)

oregano, fresh (1 bunch)

parsley, fresh (1 bunch)

raspberries (½ cup)

red bell peppers (8)

red onions (3)

scallions (3)

spinach (1 cup)

strawberries (1½ cups)

sweet onions (5)

thyme, fresh (2 bunches)

tomatoes (6)

zucchini (10)

CANNED AND BOTTLED ITEMS

chicken broth, low-sodium (2½ cups)

chickpeas, sodium-free (4 [15-ounce] cans)

Dijon mustard (4 teaspoons)

extra-virgin olive oil (2 cups)

navy beans, sodium-free
(2 [15-ounce] cans)

olive oil nonstick cooking spray

pumpkin purée (1¼ cups)

vegetable broth, sodium-free (4 cups)

Worcestershire sauce (4 teaspoons)

PANTRY ITEMS

allspice, ground

almond flour

almonds, chopped

baking powder

baking soda

balsamic vinegar

black pepper

bread crumbs

chili powder

cinnamon, ground

coconut oil

coriander, ground

cumin, ground

garlic powder

granulated sweetener

honey

nutmeg, ground

paprika, smoked

pine nuts

quinoa

sea salt

vanilla extract

whole-wheat bread

whole-wheat pastry flour

whole-wheat pitas

whole-wheat tortilla wraps

WEEK 2 MEAL PLAN

MONDAY

Breakfast: Easy Breakfast Chia Pudding

Snack: 2 ounces smoked salmon, tomato slices, 1 tablespoon low-fat cream cheese on 2 high-fiber crackers

Lunch: Leftover Juicy Turkey Burger on a whole-wheat bun, and Sautéed Mixed Vegetables

Snack: ½ ounce dark chocolate

Dinner: Pork Chop Diane, and Zucchini Noodles with Lime Basil Pesto (double the recipes so you'll have leftovers for tomorrow)

Total Carbs Per Day: 143g

TUESDAY

Breakfast: Spanakopita Egg White Frittata with 1 slice whole-wheat toast

Snack: ¼ cup hummus, and 1 ounce whole-grain pretzels

Lunch: Leftover Pork Chop Diane, and Zucchini Noodles with Lime Basil Pesto

Snack: ½ whole-wheat English muffin, and ⅛ avocado

Dinner: Herb-Crusted Halibut, and Whole-Wheat Couscous with Pecans (double the recipes so you'll have leftovers for tomorrow)

Total Carbs Per Day: 140g

WEDNESDAY

Breakfast: Oatmeal Strawberry Smoothie

Snack: 1 medium baked apple with cinnamon, 7 crushed walnut halves

Lunch: Leftover Herb-Crusted Halibut, and Whole-Wheat Couscous with Pecans

Snack: 1 ounce nitrate-free beef or turkey jerky

Dinner: Chicken and Roasted Vegetable Wrap, and Broiled Spinach (double the recipes so you'll have leftovers for tomorrow)

Total Carbs Per Day: 150g

THURSDAY

Breakfast: Summer Veggie Scramble, and 1 orange

Snack: ½ medium apple, and 1 teaspoon almond butter

Lunch: Leftover Chicken and Roasted Vegetable Wrap, and Broiled Spinach

Snack: 1 Cookies and Cream Quest bar

Dinner: Coffee-and-Herb-Marinated Steak, and Mediterranean Chickpea Slaw (double the recipes so you'll have leftovers for tomorrow)

Total Carbs Per Day: 146g

FRIDAY

Breakfast: Cottage Cheese Almond Pancakes with ½ cup unsweetened applesauce

Snack: 40 peanuts

Lunch: Leftover Coffee-and-Herb-Marinated Steak, and Mediterranean Chickpea Slaw

Snack: ½ ounce low-fat cheese, and ½ ounce whole-grain crackers

Dinner: Tabbouleh Pita, and Nutmeg Green Beans

Total Carbs Per Day: 145g

SATURDAY

Breakfast: Fruity Avocado Smoothie, and 1 slice whole-wheat toast spread with 1 tablespoon almond butter

Snack: ½ cup low-fat cottage cheese, and 1 medium peach

Lunch: Wild Mushroom Frittata with 1 sliced tomato

Snack: 1 So Delicious Coconutmilk Dairy-Free Frozen Dessert Fudge Bar Mini

Dinner: Lime-Parsley Lamb Cutlets, and Barley Squash Risotto (double the recipes so you'll have leftovers for tomorrow)

Total Carbs Per Day: 150g

SUNDAY

Breakfast: Creamy Green Smoothie

Snack: 15 baked tortilla chips, and 3 tablespoons guacamole

Lunch: Leftover Lime-Parsley Lamb Cutlets, and Barley Squash Risotto

Snack: 1 small piece fruit (such as apple, orange, peach), and 1 ounce part-skim string cheese

Dinner: Orange-Infused Scallops, and Whole-Wheat Linguine with Kale Pesto

Total Carbs Per Day: 140g

WEEK 2 SHOPPING LIST

MEAT AND SEAFOOD

chicken breasts, boneless, skinless
(4 [8 ounce])

flank steak (2 pounds)

halibut fillets (8 [5 ounce])

lamb cutlets (24 [about 3 pounds total])

pork top loin chops, boneless (8 [5 ounce])

sea scallops (2 pounds)

DAIRY, DAIRY ALTERNATIVES, AND EGGS

almond milk, unsweetened, plain (7 cups)

butter (2½ tablespoons)

cottage cheese, low-fat (2 cups)

eggs (30)

feta cheese, low-sodium (1½ cups)

goat cheese (½ cup)

Greek yogurt, 2 percent, plain (¼ cup)

milk, skim (3½ cups)

Parmesan cheese (2 ounces)

PRODUCE

apple, Granny Smith (1)

avocado (1)

banana (1)

basil, fresh (3 bunches)

blueberries (½ cup)

butternut squash (1)

PRODUCE *continued*

cherry tomatoes (2 cups)

chives, fresh (1 bunch)

eggplant (1)

English cucumbers (3)

garlic, (1 head)

green beans (1½ pounds)

kale (2 bunches)

lemons (2)

limes (8)

mushrooms, cremini, oyster, shiitake, portobello, etc. (2 cups)

oranges (2)

oregano, fresh (1 bunch)

parsley, fresh (2 bunches)

red bell peppers (5)

red onions (2)

rosemary, fresh (1 bunch)

scallions (5)

spinach (19 cups)

strawberries, frozen (1 cup)

sweet onions (2)

thyme, fresh (2 bunches)

tomatoes (4)

yellow bell peppers (2)

zucchini (11)

CANNED AND BOTTLED ITEMS

almond butter (1 tablespoon)

applesauce, unsweetened (½ cup)

chicken broth, low-sodium (½ cup)

chickpeas packed in water
(2 [15-ounce] cans)

Dijon mustard (4 teaspoons)

olive oil nonstick cooking spray

sun-dried tomatoes (½ cup)

Worcestershire sauce (4 teaspoons)

PANTRY ITEMS

almond flour

almonds, chopped

apple cider vinegar

balsamic vinegar

barley

black pepper

bulgur wheat

chia seeds

cinnamon, ground

coffee beans, whole

cumin, ground

honey

nutmeg, ground

oats

olive oil

pecans, chopped

pine nuts

pistachios

sea salt

vanilla extract

whole-wheat bread

whole-wheat couscous

whole-wheat linguine

whole-wheat pitas

whole-wheat tortilla wraps

1,800-CALORIE WEEKLY MEAL PLANS AND SHOPPING LISTS

WEEK 1 MEAL PLAN

MONDAY

Breakfast: Easy Breakfast Chia Pudding with 1 cup sliced strawberries, and 2 tablespoons sunflower seeds

Snack: 1 Kind Dark Chocolate, Nuts and Sea Salt bar

Lunch: Chicken and Roasted Vegetable Wrap, and Broiled Spinach

Snack: 23 to 25 pistachios

Dinner: Spicy Citrus Sole, and Barley Squash Risotto, and Wilted Kale and Chard (double the recipes so you'll have leftovers for tomorrow)

Total Carbs Per Day: 180g

TUESDAY

Breakfast: Summer Veggie Scramble with 2 slices whole-wheat toast

Snack: 16 to 18 cashew halves

Lunch: Leftover Spicy Citrus Sole, and Barley Squash Risotto, and Wilted Kale and Chard

Snack: 3 tablespoons guacamole, and 1 cup assorted raw vegetables

Dinner: Lime-Parsley Lamb Cutlets, and Mediterranean Chickpea Slaw (double the recipes so you'll have leftovers for tomorrow)

Total Carbs Per Day: 167g

WEDNESDAY

Breakfast: Cottage Cheese Almond Pancakes with 1 cup raspberries

Snack: ½ cup blueberries, 6 ounces 2 percent plain Greek yogurt, and 1 tablespoon sunflower seeds

Lunch: Leftover Lime-Parsley Lamb Cutlets, and Mediterranean Chickpea Slaw

Snack: 1 Enlightened Ice Cream bar

Dinner: Tantalizing Jerked Chicken, and Zucchini Noodles with Lime-Basil Pesto (double the recipes so you'll have leftovers for tomorrow)

Total Carbs Per Day: 165g

THURSDAY

Breakfast: 2 Lemon Blueberry Muffins with 1 tablespoon butter

Snack: 15 baked tortilla chips, and 3 tablespoons guacamole

Lunch: Leftover Tantalizing Jerked Chicken, and Zucchini Noodles with Lime-Basil Pesto

Snack: ½ small whole-wheat pita (½ ounce), and ½ ounce low-fat cheese spread

Dinner: Coffee-and-Herb-Marinated Steak, and Quinoa Vegetable Skillet, and Roasted Eggplant with Goat Cheese (double the recipes so you'll have leftovers for tomorrow)

Total Carbs Per Day: 171g

FRIDAY

Breakfast: Spanakopita Egg White Frittata, 1 toasted whole-wheat English muffin spread with 1 tablespoon butter, and 1 orange

Snack: 1 medium baked apple with cinnamon, 7 crushed walnut halves

Lunch: Leftover Coffee-and-Herb-Marinated Steak, and Quinoa Vegetable Skillet, and Roasted Eggplant with Goat Cheese

Snack: ¼ cup pomegranate seeds, and 4 ounces 2 percent plain Greek yogurt

Dinner: Juicy Turkey Burgers on a whole-grain bun, and Sautéed Mixed Vegetables (double the recipes so you'll have leftovers for tomorrow)

Total Carbs Per Day: 170g

SATURDAY

Breakfast: 2 Lemon Blueberry Muffins with 1 tablespoon butter

Snack: 1 medium banana, and 1 tablespoon peanut butter

Lunch: Leftover Juicy Turkey Burgers on a whole-grain bun, and Sautéed Mixed Vegetables

Snack: ½ medium apple, and 1 teaspoon almond butter

Dinner: Orange-Infused Scallops, and Pico de Gallo Navy Beans, and Asparagus with Cashews (double the recipes, except the asparagus)

Total Carbs Per Day: 175g

SUNDAY

Breakfast: Greek Yogurt Cinnamon Pancakes with 1 tablespoon butter, and 1 cup blueberries

Snack: 23 to 25 pistachios

Lunch: Leftover Orange-Infused Scallops, and Pico de Gallo Navy Beans

Snack: ½ cup Breyer's No Sugar Added Vanilla Bean ice cream

Dinner: Pork Chop Diane, and Whole-Wheat Couscous with Pecans, and Nutmeg Green Beans (double the recipes so you'll have leftovers for tomorrow)

Total Carbs Per Day: 180g

WEEK 1 SHOPPING LIST

MEAT AND SEAFOOD

chicken breasts, boneless, skinless
(2 [8 ounce] and 8 [5 ounce])

flank steak (2 pounds)

ground turkey (3 pounds)

lamb cutlets (24 [about 3 pounds total])

pork top loin chops, boneless (8 [5 ounce])

sea scallops (4 pounds)

sole fillets (8 [6 ounce])

DAIRY, DAIRY ALTERNATIVES, AND EGGS

almond milk, unsweetened plain (4 cups)

butter (½ cup plus 1 teaspoon)

cottage cheese, low-fat (2 cups)

eggs (19)

feta cheese, low-fat (2½ cups)

Greek yogurt, 2 percent, plain (1¾ cups)

milk, skim (1 cup)

PRODUCE

asparagus (2 pounds)

basil, fresh (4 bunches)

blueberries (3 cups)

broccoli (2 heads)

butternut squash (1)

carrots (6)

cauliflower (2 heads)

cherry tomatoes (2 cups)

PRODUCE *continued*

chives, fresh (1 bunch)

eggplants (3)

English cucumbers (2)

garlic (1 head)

green beans (4 pounds)

habanero chile peppers (4)

jalapeño pepper (1)

kale (3 pounds)

lemons (4)

limes (10)

oranges (3)

oregano, fresh (1 bunch)

parsley, fresh (2 bunches)

raspberries (1 cup)

red bell peppers (7)

red onion (1)

rosemary, fresh (1 bunch)

scallions (6)

spinach (10 cups)

strawberries (1 cup)

sweet onions (5)

Swiss chard (2 pounds)

thyme, fresh (2 bunches)

tomatoes (5)

yellow bell pepper (1)

zucchini (11)

CANNED AND BOTTLED ITEMS

chicken broth, low-sodium (½ cup)

chickpeas packed in water
(2 [15-ounce] cans)

corn kernels (2 cups)

Dijon mustard (4 teaspoons)

navy beans, sodium-free
(2 [15-ounce] cans)

Worcestershire sauce (4 teaspoons)

PANTRY ITEMS

allspice, ground

almond flour

apple cider vinegar

baking powder

baking soda

balsamic vinegar

barley

black pepper

bread crumbs

bulgur wheat

cardamom, ground

cashews

chia seeds

chili powder

cinnamon, ground

cloves, ground

coconut oil

PANTRY ITEMS *continued*

coffee beans, whole

coriander, ground

cumin, ground

extra-virgin olive oil

garlic powder

granulated sweetener

honey

nutmeg, ground

oats

olive oil nonstick cooking spray

paprika, smoked

pecans

pine nuts

pistachios

quinoa

sea salt

sunflower seeds

vanilla extract

vegetable broth, low-sodium

whole-wheat bread

whole-wheat couscous

whole-wheat English muffin

whole-wheat pastry flour

whole-wheat pitas

whole-wheat tortilla wraps

WEEK 2 MEAL PLAN

MONDAY

Breakfast: Sweet Quinoa Cereal, and Plum Smoothie

Snack: 8 or 9 cashew halves

Lunch: Leftover Pork Chop Diane, and Whole-Wheat Couscous with Pecans, and Nutmeg Green Beans

Snack: ½ ounce low-fat cheese, and ½ ounce whole-grain crackers

Dinner: Herb-Crusted Halibut, and Whole-Wheat Linguine with Kale Pesto, and Wilted Kale and Chard (double the recipes so you'll have leftovers for tomorrow)

Total Carbs Per Day: 180g

TUESDAY

Breakfast: 2 Bran Apple Muffins with 1 tablespoon almond butter

Snack: ½ ounce dark chocolate

Lunch: Leftover Herb-Crusted Halibut, and Whole-Wheat Linguine with Kale Pesto, and Wilted Kale and Chard

Snack: 3 tablespoons hummus, and 1 cup assorted raw vegetables

Dinner: Tabbouleh Pita, and Pico de Gallo Navy Beans

Total Carb Per Day: 180g

WEDNESDAY

Breakfast: Cottage Cheese Almond Pancakes with 1 sliced peach

Snack: 10 to 12 almonds

Lunch: Chicken and Roasted Vegetable Wrap

Snack: 2 ounces smoked salmon, tomato slices, 1 tablespoon low-fat cream cheese on 2 high-fiber crackers

Dinner: Coffee-and-Herb-Marinated Steak, and Fennel and Chickpeas, and Golden Lemony Wax Beans (double the recipes, except the wax beans)

Total Carbs Per Day: 180g

THURSDAY

Breakfast: 2 Bran Apple Muffins with 1 tablespoon butter, and ½ cantaloupe

Snack: ¼ cup hummus, and 1 ounce whole-grain pretzels

Lunch: Mediterranean Steak Sandwich (using leftover Coffee-and-Herb-Marinated Steak), and leftover Fennel and Chickpeas

Snack: ½ ounce dark chocolate

Dinner: Juicy Turkey Burger, and Quinoa Vegetable Skillet, and Broiled Spinach (double the recipes, except the spinach)

Total Carbs Per Day: 180g

FRIDAY

Breakfast: Wild Mushroom Frittata, 2 slices whole-wheat toast spread with 2 teaspoons butter, and 1 cup sliced strawberries

Snack: 1 Cookies and Cream Quest bar

Lunch: Leftover Juicy Turkey Burger, and Quinoa Vegetable Skillet

Snack: 1 small fruit (apple, orange, peach, etc.), and 1 ounce part-skim string cheese

Dinner: Chipotle Chili Pork Chops, and Zucchini Noodles with Lime-Basil Pesto (double the recipes so you'll have leftovers for tomorrow)

Total Carbs Per Day: 165g

SATURDAY

Breakfast: Easy Breakfast Chia Pudding with 2 tablespoons chopped almonds, and ½ cup raspberries, Carrot Pear Smoothie

Snack: 1 Cookies and Cream Quest bar

Lunch: Leftover Chipotle Chili Pork Chops, and Zucchini Noodles with Lime-Basil Pesto

Snack: 1 So Delicious Coconutmilk Dairy-Free Frozen Dessert Fudge Bar Mini

Dinner: Sole Piccata, and Barley Squash Risotto, and Sautéed Mixed Vegetables (double the recipes so you'll have leftovers for tomorrow)

Total Carbs Per Day: 179g

SUNDAY

Breakfast: Greek Yogurt Cinnamon Pancakes with 1 tablespoon butter, and Plum Smoothie

Snack: ½ medium apple, and 1 teaspoon almond butter

Lunch: Leftover Sole Piccata, and Barley Squash Risotto, and Sautéed Mixed Vegetables

Snack: ½ cup low-fat cottage cheese, 1 small peach

Dinner: Tantalizing Jerked Chicken, and Mediterranean Chickpea Slaw

Total Carbs Per Day: 180g

WEEK 2 SHOPPING LIST

MEAT AND SEAFOOD

chicken breasts, boneless, skinless
(2 [8 ounce] and 4 [5 ounce])

flank steak (2 pounds)

ground turkey (3 pounds)

halibut fillets (8 [5 ounce])

pork chops (8 [5 ounce])

sole fillets (8 [5 ounce])

DAIRY, DAIRY ALTERNATIVES, AND EGGS

eggs (19)

almond milk, unsweetened, plain (4 cups)

butter (¾ cup)

cottage cheese, low-fat (2 cups)

feta cheese, low-sodium (5 ounces)

goat cheese (½ cup)

Greek yogurt, 2 percent, plain (14 ounces)

milk, skim (4 cups)

Parmesan cheese (4 ounces)

PRODUCE

apples (2)

basil, fresh (5 bunches)

broccoli (2 heads)

butternut squash (1)

cantaloupe (1)

carrots (8)

cauliflower (2 heads)

cherry tomatoes (3 cups)

corn kernels, fresh or frozen (2 cups)

eggplant (1)

PRODUCE *continued*

English cucumber (1)

fennel bulbs (2)

garlic (1 head)

green beans (2 cups)

habanero chile peppers (2)

jalapeño pepper (1)

kale (4 pounds)

lemons (4)

lettuce (1 head)

limes (8)

mushrooms, cremini, oyster, shiitake, portobello, etc. (2 cups)

oregano, fresh (1 bunch)

parsley, fresh (1 bunch)

peach (1)

plums (8)

raspberries (½ cup)

red bell peppers (6)

red onions (2)

rosemary, fresh (1 bunch)

scallions (3)

strawberries (1½ cups)

sweet onions (6)

Swiss chard (2 pounds)

thyme, fresh (2 bunches)

tomatoes (3)

wax beans (2 pounds)

yellow bell pepper (1)

zucchini (10)

CANNED AND BOTTLED ITEMS

almond butter (1 tablespoon)

capers (4 tablespoons)

chicken broth, low sodium (6 cups)

chickpeas, sodium-free (3 [15-ounce] cans)

navy beans, sodium-free (1 [15-ounce] can)

sun-dried tomatoes (1 cup)

vegetable broth, low-sodium (4 cups)

PANTRY ITEMS

allspice, ground

almond flour

almonds, chopped

apple cider vinegar

baking powder

balsamic vinegar

barley

black pepper

bulgur wheat

cardamom, ground

chia seeds

chipotle chili powder

cinnamon, ground

cloves, ground

coconut oil

PANTRY ITEMS *continued*

coffee beans, whole

coriander, ground

cumin, ground

extra-virgin olive oil

flour, all-purpose

ginger, ground

granulated sweetener

nutmeg, ground

oats

olive oil nonstick cooking spray

pine nuts

pistachios

quinoa

sea salt

vanilla extract

wheat bran

whole-wheat bread

whole-wheat breadcrumbs

whole-wheat flour

whole-wheat linguine

whole-wheat pitas

whole-wheat tortilla wraps

2,100-CALORIE WEEKLY MEAL PLANS AND SHOPPING LISTS

WEEK 1 MEAL PLAN

MONDAY

Breakfast: Cottage Cheese Almond Pancakes with 1 tablespoon butter, and 1 cup sliced strawberries

Snack: 1 Cookies and Cream Quest bar

Lunch: Chicken and Roasted Vegetable Wrap with 1 sliced apple

Snack: 1 ounce beef or turkey jerky, nitrate-free

Dinner: Lime-Parsley Lamb Cutlets, and Barley Squash Risotto, and Asparagus with Cashews (double the recipes so you'll have leftovers for tomorrow)

Total Carbs Per Day: 192g

TUESDAY

Breakfast: 2 Lemon Blueberry Muffins with 2 teaspoons butter

Snack: ½ cup blueberries, 6 ounces 2 percent plain Greek yogurt, 1 tablespoon sunflower seeds

Lunch: Leftover Lime-Parsley Lamb Cutlets, and Barley Squash Risotto, and Asparagus with Cashews

Snack: 23 to 25 pistachios

Dinner: Juicy Turkey Burger on a whole-wheat bun with tomato slices, and 1 slice low-fat Swiss cheese, plus Pico de Gallo Navy Beans (double the recipes so you'll have leftovers for tomorrow)

Total Carbs Per Day: 215g

WEDNESDAY

Breakfast: Plum Smoothie

Snack: 1 Lemon Blueberry Muffin with 1 teaspoon butter

Lunch: Leftover Juicy Turkey Burger on a whole-wheat bun with tomato slices, and 1 slice low-fat Swiss cheese, plus Pico de Gallo Navy Beans

Snack: ½ medium apple, and 1 teaspoon almond butter

Dinner: Baked Salmon with Lemon Sauce, and Whole-Wheat Couscous with Pecans, and Wilted Kale and Chard (double the recipes so you'll have leftovers for tomorrow)

Total Carbs Per Day: 220g

THURSDAY

Breakfast: 2 Lemon Blueberry Muffins with 2 teaspoons butter

Snack: 40 peanuts

Lunch: Leftover Baked Salmon with Lemon Sauce, and Whole-Wheat Couscous with Pecans, and Wilted Kale and Chard

Snack: ¼ cup pomegranate seeds, and 4 ounces 2 percent plain Greek yogurt

Dinner: Coffee-and-Herb-Marinated Steak, and Whole-Wheat Linguine with Kale Pesto, and Nutmeg Green Beans (double the recipes, except the green beans)

Total Carbs Per Day: 182g

FRIDAY

Breakfast: Greek Yogurt Cinnamon Pancakes with 1 tablespoon butter, and 1 cup blueberries

Snack: 1 medium banana, and 1 tablespoon peanut butter

Lunch: Mediterranean Steak Sandwich (using leftover Coffee-and-Herb-Marinated Steak) with 1 tablespoon fat-free sour cream, and leftover Whole-Wheat Linguine with Kale Pesto

Snack: 1 small low-carb whole-wheat tortilla, and 2 tablespoons shredded mozzarella cheese

Dinner: Tantalizing Jerked Chicken, and Zucchini Noodles with Lime-Basil Pesto, and Asparagus with Cashews (double the recipes so you'll have leftovers for tomorrow)

Total Carbs Per Day: 195g

SATURDAY

Breakfast: 2 Bran Apple Muffins with 1 tablespoon butter, and 1 cup raspberries

Snack: ½ cup low-fat cottage cheese, and 1 medium peach

Lunch: Leftover Tantalizing Jerked Chicken, and Zucchini Noodles with Lime Basil Pesto, and Asparagus with Cashews

Snack: 1 Enlightened ice cream bar

Dinner: Herb-Crusted Halibut, and Quinoa Vegetable Skillet, and Fennel and Chickpeas (double the recipes so you'll have leftovers for tomorrow)

Total Carbs Per Day: 180g

SUNDAY

Breakfast: Cottage Cheese Almond Pancakes with 2 tablespoons almond butter

Snack: 1 Kind Dark Chocolate, Nuts and Sea Salt bar

Lunch: Leftover Herb-Crusted Halibut, and Quinoa Vegetable Skillet, and Fennel and Chickpeas

Snack: 1 Bran Apple Muffin with 1 teaspoon butter

Dinner: Pork Chop Diane, and Mediterranean Chickpea Slaw, and Sautéed Mixed Vegetables (double the recipes so you'll have leftovers for tomorrow)

Total Carbs Per Day: 216g

WEEK 1 SHOPPING LIST

MEAT AND SEAFOOD

chicken breasts, boneless, skinless
(2 [8 ounce] and 8 [5 ounce])

flank steak (2 pounds)

ground turkey (3 pounds)

halibut fillets (8 [5 ounce])

lamb cutlets (24 [about 3 pounds total])

pork top loin chops, boneless (8 [5 ounce])

salmon fillets (8 (5 ounce])

DAIRY, DAIRY ALTERNATIVES, AND EGGS

butter (1 cup)

cottage cheese, low-fat (4 cups)

eggs (19)

feta cheese, low-sodium (8 ounces)

Greek yogurt, 2 percent, plain (20 ounces)

milk, skim (3½ cups)

Parmesan cheese (4 ounces)

sour cream, fat-free (1 cup)

PRODUCE

apples (3)

asparagus (8 pounds)

basil, fresh (4 bunches)

blueberries (2 cups)

broccoli (2 heads)

butternut squash (1)

PRODUCE *continued*

carrots (6)

cauliflower (2 heads)

chives, fresh (1 bunch)

English cucumbers (2)

fennel bulbs (2)

garlic (1 head)

green beans (2½ pounds)

habanero chile peppers (4)

jalapeño pepper (1)

kale (4 pounds)

lemons (6)

limes (12)

oregano, fresh (1 bunch)

parsley, fresh (2 bunches)

plums (4)

raspberries (1 cup)

red bell peppers (8)

rosemary, fresh (1 bunch)

scallions (4)

strawberries (1 cup)

sweet onions (6)

Swiss chard (2 pounds)

thyme, fresh (2 bunches)

tomatoes (6)

zucchini (10)

CANNED AND BOTTLED ITEMS

almond butter (2 tablespoons)

chicken broth, low-sodium (3½ cups)

chickpeas, sodium-free (4 [15-ounce] cans)

corn kernels (2 cups)

Dijon mustard (4 teaspoons)

navy beans, sodium-free (2 [15-ounce] cans)

sun-dried tomatoes (1 cup)

vegetable broth, low-sodium (5 cups)

Worcestershire sauce (4 teaspoons)

PANTRY ITEMS

allspice, ground

almond flour

almonds, chopped

apple cider vinegar

baking powder

baking soda

balsamic vinegar

barley

black pepper

bread crumbs

cardamom, ground

cashews

cinnamon, ground

cloves, ground

PANTRY ITEMS *continued*

coconut oil

coffee beans, whole

coriander, ground

cumin, ground

extra-virgin olive oil

ginger, ground

granulated sweetener

honey

nutmeg, ground

oats

olive oil nonstick cooking spray

pecans

pine nuts

pistachios

quinoa

sea salt

vanilla extract

wheat bran

whole-wheat couscous

whole-wheat linguine

whole-wheat pastry flour

whole-wheat tortilla wraps

WEEK 2 MEAL PLAN

MONDAY

Breakfast: 2 Bran Apple Muffins with 1 tablespoon butter, and two 1-inch cubes low-fat Cheddar

Snack: 15 baked tortilla chips, and 3 tablespoons guacamole

Lunch: Leftover Pork Chop Diane, and Mediterranean Chickpea Slaw, and Sautéed Mixed Vegetables

Snack: 15 large shrimp, and 2 tablespoons cocktail sauce

Dinner: Juicy Turkey Burgers with whole-wheat bun and ¼ avocado, sliced, and Zucchini Noodles with Lime-Basil Pesto (double the recipes so you'll have leftovers for tomorrow)

Total Carbs Per Day: 190g

TUESDAY

Breakfast: Sweet Quinoa Cereal with 1 orange

Snack: 16 to 18 cashew halves

Lunch: Leftover Juicy Turkey Burgers with whole-wheat bun and ¼ avocado, sliced, and Zucchini Noodles with Lime-Basil Pesto

Snack: 3 tablespoons hummus and 1 cup assorted raw vegetables

Dinner: Sole Piccata, and Whole-Wheat Couscous with Pecans, and Wilted Kale and Chard (double the recipes so you'll have leftovers for tomorrow)

Total Carbs Per Day: 204g

WEDNESDAY

Breakfast: Pumpkin Apple Waffles with 2 tablespoons low-fat cream cheese, and ½ cup strawberries

Snack: 1 medium peach, and ½ cup low-fat cottage cheese

Lunch: Leftover Sole Piccata, and Whole-Wheat Couscous with Pecans, and Wilted Kale and Chard

Snack: ½ ounce dark chocolate

Dinner: Lime-Parsley Lamb Cutlets, and Barley Squash Risotto, and Golden Lemony Wax Beans (double the recipes so you'll have leftovers for tomorrow)

Total Carbs Per Day: 205g

THURSDAY

Breakfast: Cottage Cheese Almond Pancakes with 1 tablespoon butter and ½ cup unsweetened applesauce, and Plum Smoothie

Snack: 1 Cookies and Cream Quest bar

Lunch: Leftover Lime-Parsley Lamb Cutlets, and Barley Squash Risotto, and Golden Lemony Wax Beans

Snack: ½ small whole-wheat pita with ½ ounce low-fat cheese spread

Dinner: Baked Salmon with Lemon Sauce, and Roasted Cinnamon Celery Root, and Sautéed Mixed Vegetables (double the recipes so you'll have leftovers for tomorrow)

Total Carbs Per Day: 196g

FRIDAY

Breakfast: Wild Mushroom Frittata, and 2 slices whole-grain toast spread with 2 teaspoons butter, and Fruity Avocado Smoothie

Snack: ¼ cup hummus, and 1 ounce whole-grain pretzels

Lunch: Leftover Baked Salmon with Lemon Sauce, and Roasted Cinnamon Celery Root, and Sautéed Mixed Vegetables

Snack: ½ medium apple, and 1 teaspoon almond butter

Dinner: Coffee and Herb Marinated Steak, and Pico de Gallo Navy Beans, and Sautéed Garlicky Mushrooms (double the recipes, except the mushrooms)

Total Carbs Per Day: 198g

SATURDAY

Breakfast: 2 Lemon Blueberry Muffins with 2 teaspoons butter, and ½ cantaloupe

Snack: ½ cup blueberries, 6 ounces 2 percent plain Greek yogurt, and 1 tablespoon sunflower seeds

Lunch: Mediterranean Steak Sandwich (using the steak from Coffee and Herb Marinated Steak), and leftover Pico de Gallo Navy Beans

Snack: ½ cup Breyer's No Sugar Added Vanilla Bean ice cream

Dinner: Chipotle Chili Pork Chops, and Mediterranean Chickpea Slaw, and Asparagus with Cashews (double the recipes so you'll have leftovers for tomorrow)

Total Carbs Per Day: 210g

SUNDAY

Breakfast: Spanakopita Egg White Frittata, and 2 slices whole-grain toast spread with 1 tablespoon butter, and Creamy Green Smoothie

Snack: 2 tablespoons shelled sunflower seeds

Lunch: Leftover Chipotle Chili Pork Chops, and Mediterranean Chickpea Slaw, and Asparagus with Cashews

Snack: 1 medium banana, and 1 tablespoon peanut butter

Dinner: Chicken and Roasted Vegetable Wrap, and Fennel and Chickpeas

Total Carbs Per Day: 195g

WEEK 2 SHOPPING LIST

MEAT AND SEAFOOD

chicken breasts, boneless, skinless (2 [8 ounce])

flank steak (2 pounds)

ground turkey (3 pounds)

lamb cutlets (24 [about 3 pounds])

pork chops (8 [5 ounce])

salmon fillets (8 [5 ounce])

sole fillets (8 [5 ounce])

DAIRY, DAIRY ALTERNATIVES, AND EGGS

almond milk, unsweetened, plain (3 cups)

butter (1 cup)

Cheddar, low-fat (1 ounce)

cottage cheese, low-fat (2 cups)

cream cheese, low-fat (5 tablespoons)

eggs (28)

feta cheese, low-sodium (11 ounces)

goat cheese (½ cup)

Greek yogurt, 2 percent, plain (18 ounces)

milk, skim (6 cups)

sour cream, fat-free (1 cup)

PRODUCE

apples (3)

asparagus (4 pounds)

avocado (4)

banana (1)

basil, fresh (4 bunches)

blueberries (1½ cups)

PRODUCE *continued*

broccoli (2 heads)

butternut squash (1)

button mushrooms (2 pounds)

cantaloupe (1)

carrots (6)

cauliflower (2 heads)

celery roots (4 [about 2 pounds])

chives, fresh (1 bunch)

eggplant (1)

English cucumbers (2)

fennel bulb (1)

garlic (1 head)

ginger, fresh (1 [3-inch] piece)

green beans (1 pound)

jalapeño pepper (1)

kale (3 pounds)

lemons (8)

lettuce (1 head)

limes (11)

mushrooms, cremini, oyster, shiitake, portobello, etc. (2 cups)

orange (1)

oregano, fresh (1 bunch)

parsley, fresh (1 bunch)

plums (4)

red bell peppers (7)

red onions (2)

rosemary, fresh (1 bunch)

scallions (4)

PRODUCE *(continued)*

spinach (11 cups)

strawberries (1½ cups)

sweet onions (4)

Swiss chard (2 pounds)

thyme, fresh (2 bunches)

tomatoes (5)

wax beans (4 pounds)

zucchini (9)

CANNED AND BOTTLED ITEMS

applesauce, unsweetened (½ cup)

capers (¼ cup)

chicken broth, low-sodium (6 cups)

chickpeas, sodium-free (3 [15-ounce] cans)

navy beans, sodium-free
(2 [15-ounce] cans)

pumpkin purée (1¼ cups)

PANTRY ITEMS

almond flour

almonds, chopped

apple cider vinegar

baking powder

baking soda

balsamic vinegar

barley

black pepper

bread crumbs

cardamom, ground

PANTRY ITEMS *continued*

cashews, chopped

chipotle chili powder

cinnamon, ground

coconut oil

coffee beans, whole

coriander, ground

cumin, ground

extra-virgin olive oil

flour, all-purpose

ginger, ground

granulated sweetener

honey

nutmeg, ground

olive oil nonstick cooking spray

pecans, chopped

pine nuts

pistachios, chopped

quinoa

sea salt

vanilla extract

wheat bran

whole-wheat bread

whole-wheat couscous

whole-wheat flour

whole-wheat pastry flour

whole-wheat pitas

whole-wheat tortilla wraps

Month Two

Now it's time to focus on other important areas of diabetes self-care, such as exercise. Regular physical activity plays a major role in blood sugar management, weight control, and overall health. It is not always easy to come up with a plan, so we will give you tips on the best kinds of exercise to do and practical suggestions to get started. If you have not been exercising, don't worry—we'll start slow with baby steps. Stress can affect blood sugar too, so you will get plenty of tips on how to decrease stress.

We also loosen up with the meal plans. While you still get specific recipes, we also provide suggestions (such as a turkey sandwich on whole-grain bread) to help you start planning meals on your own. This is a good time to practice planning your own meals. You can use the tools we talked about in chapter 1: the Plate Method or Carbohydrate Counting. Fill half your plate with vegetables, a quarter with a protein, and a quarter with a starch. Or practice Carbohydrate Counting. You can also use the On the Fly suggestions (page 38) as a guide. The goal for this month is for you to feel more comfortable planning your own meals, using our meal plans and recipes as a guide, as well as to be more active . . . and less stressed!

WEEK 1 MEAL PLANS

MONDAY

Breakfast: Egg-Stuffed Tomatoes

Snack: ½ cup blueberries, and 6 ounces 2 percent plain Greek yogurt, and 1 tablespoon sunflower seeds

Lunch: Chicken and Roasted Vegetable Wraps

Snack: 1 banana

Dinner: Vegetarian Three-Bean Chili (double the recipe so you'll have leftovers for tomorrow)

TUESDAY

Breakfast: Sweet Quinoa Cereal

Snack: ¼ cup pomegranate seeds, and 4 ounces 2 percent plain Greek yogurt

Lunch: Leftover Vegetarian Three-Bean Chili

Snack: 1 So Delicious Coconutmilk Dairy-Free Frozen Dessert Fudge Bar Mini

Dinner: Roasted Beef with Peppercorn Sauce

WEDNESDAY

Breakfast: Oatmeal with skim milk, strawberries, and chopped almonds

Snack: 1 Cookies and Cream Quest bar

Lunch: Wild Mushroom Frittata

Snack: ½ medium apple, and 1 teaspoon almond butter

Dinner: Autumn Pork Chops with Red Cabbage and Apples

THURSDAY

Breakfast: Summer Veggie Scramble

Snack: ½ small whole-wheat pita, and ½ ounce low-fat cheese spread

Lunch: Turkey Cabbage Soup (double the recipe so you'll have leftovers for tomorrow)

Snack: ½ ounce dark chocolate

Dinner: Pork Chop Diane

FRIDAY

Breakfast: 2 scrambled eggs with 1 piece whole-grain toast spread with 1 teaspoon butter, and 1 cup raspberries

Snack: 40 peanuts

Lunch: Leftover Turkey Cabbage Soup

Snack: 15 baked tortilla chips, and 3 tablespoons guacamole

Dinner: Lime-Parsley Lamb Cutlets

SATURDAY

Breakfast: Cottage Cheese Almond Pancakes

Snack: 16 to 18 cashew halves

Lunch: Mediterranean Steak Sandwiches

Snack: 1 ounce beef or turkey jerky, nitrate-free

Dinner: Herb-Roasted Turkey and Vegetable (double the recipe so you'll have leftovers for tomorrow)

SUNDAY

Breakfast: Ratatouille Baked Eggs (double the ratatouille)

Snack: ¼ cup hummus, and 1 ounce whole-grain pretzels

Lunch: Leftover Herb-Roasted Turkey and Vegetables

Snack: 23 to 25 pistachios

Dinner: Coconut Chicken Curry

WEEK 2 MEAL PLAN

MONDAY

Breakfast: Simple Buckwheat Porridge

Snack: 23 to 25 pistachios

Lunch: Leftover Ratatouille

Snack: ¼ cup pomegranate seeds, and 4 ounces 2 percent plain Greek yogurt

Dinner: 1 6-ounce salmon fillet, ½ cup quinoa, and 1 cup sautéed vegetables

TUESDAY

Breakfast: 6 ounces 2 percent plain Greek yogurt with 2 tablespoons pumpkin seeds and ½ cup strawberries, and 1 toasted whole-wheat English muffin

Snack: ½ medium apple, and 1 teaspoon almond butter

Lunch: Beef Barley Soup

Snack: 1 So Delicious Coconutmilk Dairy-Free Frozen Dessert Fudge Bar Mini

Dinner: Vegetable Kale Lasagna (double the recipe so you'll have leftovers for tomorrow)

WEDNESDAY

Breakfast: Egg-Stuffed Tomatoes

Snack: 1 banana

Lunch: Leftover Vegetable Kale Lasagna

Snack: ½ small whole-wheat pita, and ½ ounce low-fat cheese spread

Dinner: Chicken tacos with a whole-wheat tortilla, filled with shredded cooked chicken, tomatoes, lettuce, fresh cilantro, and black beans

THURSDAY

Breakfast: Pumpkin Apple Waffles

Snack: 15 baked tortilla chips, and 3 tablespoons guacamole

Lunch: Seafood Stew

Snack: 1 Cookies and Cream Quest bar

Dinner: Juicy Turkey Burgers (double the recipe so you'll have leftovers for tomorrow)

FRIDAY

Breakfast: Spicy Tomato Smoothie

Snack: ½ ounce dark chocolate

Lunch: Leftover Juicy Turkey Burgers

Snack: 1 ounce beef or turkey jerky, nitrate-free

Dinner: 1 cup whole-grain pasta with 1 tablespoon pesto, 1 cup mixed vegetables, and 1 tablespoon grated Parmesan cheese

SATURDAY

Breakfast: 2 Lemon Blueberry Muffins

Snack: ¼ cup hummus, and 1 ounce whole-grain pretzels

Lunch: Tomato Baked Beans

Snack: 40 peanuts

Dinner: Crab Cakes with Honeydew Melon Salsa

SUNDAY

Breakfast: Wild Mushroom Frittata

Snack: ½ cup blueberries, and 6 ounces 2 percent plain Greek yogurt with 1 tablespoon sunflower seeds

Lunch: Creamy Mac and Cheese

Snack: 9 cashews

Dinner: Roasted 6-ounce chicken breast, brown rice, and sautéed broccoli

ACTIVITY PLAN

Regular physical activity plays a vital part in diabetes management as it increases your sensitivity to insulin. This is important, because most people with type 2 diabetes are insulin resistant. Exercise can also lower blood sugar—even hours after you exercise.

There are two main types of exercise: aerobic (which gets the heart pumping) and strength training (which involves weights and resistance). They both have health benefits and play important roles in diabetes management. An exercise program that includes aerobic and strength training burns calories and builds muscle, which helps you lose weight and keep it off.

There are even more good reasons to exercise. Regular exercise will:

+ decrease your risk of heart disease and stroke
+ lower cholesterol and blood pressure
+ strengthen bones
+ aid in weight loss and maintenance
+ improve balance
+ ease joint pain from arthritis
+ improve mood, memory, and mental health
+ help you sleep better
+ relieve stress
+ slow loss of muscle mass
+ increase your energy for daily activities

Always check with your doctor before starting any exercise program to make sure the exercise you have chosen is right for you. In addition, insulin and certain medications can increase the risk for low blood sugar (hypoglycemia). Your doctor or dietitian can give you advice on this. The following exercise recommendations are from the American Diabetes Association.

Aerobic Exercise

Aerobic exercise is any kind of exercise that gets the heart rate up. Examples include brisk walking, jogging, biking, dancing, Zumba, kickboxing, swimming, water aerobics, using a stair climber or elliptical machine, skiing, and hiking.

Recommendations

Aim for 30 minutes, five times a week, or 150 minutes a week of moderate to vigorous intensity aerobic exercise. (Moderate intensity means you are working hard enough that you can talk but not sing during the activity. Vigorous intensity means you cannot say more than a few words without pausing for a breath during the activity.) Spread your activity out over at least three days during the week, and try not to go more than two days in a row without exercising. If you are trying to lose weight and keep it off, most people need to do closer to 60 minutes of aerobic exercise a day.

Tips to get started

If you are just starting out, take it slow. Begin with 5 to 10 minutes a day and slowly build up. You don't have to do 30 minutes all at once; you can break it up into shorter sessions throughout the day. For example, you could take a 10-minute walk after each meal. You'll still get the benefits.

Strength Training

Strength training means using your muscles to work against the resistance of something like weights. Many of my patients with type 2 diabetes neglect strength training (also known as resistance training). However, this type of exercise is very important for diabetes management. Studies have shown it significantly increases insulin sensitivity and lowers blood glucose. The combination of aerobic and strength training has the greatest effect on lowering HbA1c (a measure of what your average blood sugar levels have been over a period of weeks or months). Strength training also helps with weight loss; the more muscle you have, the more calories you burn, even when you are at rest.

Recommendations

Aim to do strength training at least twice a week, in addition to your aerobic exercise. Use free weights, weight machines, or resistance bands (large, stretchy bands that look like giant rubber bands). Each session should consist of at least five or more different resistance exercises that involve the large muscle groups.

Tips to get started

Use DVDs (look in your local library) or YouTube or other online videos for weight-training workouts. If you are just starting out, look for videos for beginners. You can also check out on-demand strength training exercise videos. Go to a local YMCA, health club, or senior center for strength training classes. Or consider working with a qualified personal trainer, for even a few sessions, to learn proper technique. Other activities, such as heavy gardening, also build and maintain muscle.

Less Sedentary Time

It's estimated that we spend more than half of our waking hours sitting. Think about it—how many hours do you spend sitting a day? Most of us sit when we are at work, when we watch television, when we are on the computer, when we eat, etc. Too much "sitting time" has been linked to increased risk of heart disease, type 2 diabetes, cancer, and possibly dementia. Research suggests it may also result in higher blood sugar levels. The exact mechanism is unclear, but sitting too long may affect the way we process fats and glucose.

Recommendations

All individuals, including those with type 2 diabetes, should be encouraged to reduce the amount of time spent sitting for extended periods of time. Every 60 to 90 minutes you should stand up and move for a few minutes. Even if you exercise daily, but still sit for extended periods of time, you are at an increased risk. Newer guidelines by the American Diabetes Association recommend that prolonged sitting should be interrupted with bouts of light activity every 30 minutes for blood glucose benefits, at least in adults with type 2 diabetes.

Tips to get started

Stand up and march in place during TV commercials. Set an alarm on your smartphone or fitness tracker to buzz once an hour to remind you to get up. Alternate working at a sitting desk with a standing desk. Have a standing meeting at work. Stand when making phone calls. Take the stairs instead of elevators at work.

Sticking with It

Once you've decided it's time for a change, it's easy to start an exercise routine. But keeping it up can be a challenge. Here are some tips to help you stick to your exercise program.

+ Keep a log of when you exercise. Set a goal each week and check it off when you meet it. Writing things down can make you feel more motivated (and accountable!).

+ Find an exercise buddy. It can be helpful if someone is there to keep you on track to do the workouts you say you'll do. Exercise can even become a social time.

+ Sign up for an event like a local charity walk or run.

+ Get a fitness tracker like Fitbit, Jawbone, Apple Watch, or Garmin Vivofit. Set a goal for steps and increase it a little each week.

+ Sign up for a challenge. Many workplaces offer a steps challenge. You can also find challenges online. You can set up challenges with your friends, using many of the fitness trackers, too.

+ Find an activity you like. It's easier to maintain your commitment if you actually look forward to your active time.

+ Buy a new exercise outfit. You likely don't want to put on the same old threadbare sweatpants. Removing any possible barriers to actually getting your exercise done, however trivial they might seem, will make it easier to stick with the habit.

+ Sign up for series of classes like Zumba, kickboxing, or yoga.

+ Plan your workouts ahead of time. Thinking that you'll "get around to" working out is a sure way to end up at the gym without your running shoes. Planning ahead to do a specific activity at a specific time ensures that you'll think through everything you need, and you'll be less likely to let other obligations get in the way of your workout.

+ Try new activities to avoid boredom.

STRESS MANAGEMENT PLAN

Life can be stressful, and being diagnosed with diabetes can make you feel even more stressed. This becomes a vicious cycle because when you feel stressed, you are less likely to stick to a healthy eating and exercise plan. High levels of stress can raise blood sugar. Raised blood sugar levels can impair sound thinking and decision making, which can cause you to feel strong negative emotions. And prolonged high levels of stress can have serious negative consequences on almost every system in your body, including your cardiovascular and immune systems.

It is really important to find ways to manage your stress. Here are a few helpful stress-management tips.

*   Regular physical activity: Find an activity that you enjoy or that challenges you. Exercising to music can also be beneficial.

*   Yoga, meditation, and breathing exercises: There are even some meditation apps that can guide you, such as Headspace, Buddhify, and Calm.

*   Do mini-meditation exercises when you feel stressed. Close your eyes for five minutes, try to clear your mind, and focus on your breathing.

*   Replace negative thoughts with positive ones. Whenever a negative thought pops into your mind, immediately change your thought process and think of something positive.

*   Make time to do the things you want to do for yourself, whether it is getting a manicure, spending time with your children or grandchildren, playing golf with the guys, or watching your favorite television show.

*   Think of three positive things every day.

Month Three

This month is all about your wellness plan. The focus shifts to issues like maintaining your emotional health and dealing with social challenges. We will continue to help you by suggesting recipes for meal planning, but by now you should be feeling more confident about making healthy food choices, selecting the right portion sizes, and balancing your meals throughout the day.

Because diabetes is a lifelong condition, keeping yourself emotionally healthy is just as important as the physical aspect. We discuss some of the common challenges that people with diabetes may face, such as feeling overwhelmed, depressed, or having to deal with checking blood sugar. In addition, we give you practical tips on handling social challenges like restaurant dining, parties, and holidays.

WEEK 1 MEAL PLANS

MONDAY

Breakfast: 1 scrambled egg, 1 piece whole-grain toast spread with 1 teaspoon butter, and 1 cup strawberries

Lunch: Chicken and Roasted Vegetable Wrap

Dinner: Red Lentil Soup (double the recipe so you'll have leftovers for tomorrow)

TUESDAY

Breakfast: Egg-Stuffed Tomatoes

Lunch: Leftover Red Lentil Soup

Dinner: 1 (6-ounce) roasted chicken breast, brown rice, and sautéed broccoli

WEDNESDAY

Breakfast: Tzatziki Smoothie

Lunch: Beef Barley Soup

Dinner: 1 (6-ounce) salmon fillet, ½ cup quinoa, and 1 cup sautéed green beans

THURSDAY

Breakfast: 6 ounces 2 percent plain Greek yogurt with 2 tablespoons pumpkin seeds and ½ cup strawberries, and 1 toasted whole-wheat English muffin

Lunch: Turkey Cabbage Soup (double the recipe so you'll have leftovers for tomorrow)

Dinner: 1 cup whole-grain pasta with 1 tablespoon pesto, 1 cup mixed vegetables, and 1 tablespoon grated Parmesan cheese

FRIDAY

Breakfast: Vanilla Steel-Cut Oatmeal

Lunch: Leftover Turkey Cabbage Soup

Dinner: Vegetarian Three-Bean Chili (double the recipe so you'll have leftovers for tomorrow)

SATURDAY

Breakfast: 2-egg omelet with 1 ounce shredded low-fat Cheddar cheese, and 1 slice toasted whole-grain bread spread with 1 teaspoon almond butter

Lunch: Leftover Vegetarian Three-Bean Chili

Dinner: Spicy Chicken Cacciatore (double the recipe so you'll have leftovers for tomorrow)

SUNDAY

Breakfast: 2 sunny-side up eggs with sliced tomato, and ½ cantaloupe

Lunch: Leftover Spicy Chicken Cacciatore

Dinner: Autumn Pork Chops with Red Cabbage and Apples

WEEK 2 MEAL PLAN

MONDAY

Breakfast: Broccoli Cheese Breakfast Casserole

Lunch: Tuna salad made with canned tuna, light mayo, diced celery, lemon juice, and freshly ground black pepper, served on whole-grain bread, and 1 apple on the side

Dinner: Vegetable Kale Lasagna (double the recipe so you'll have leftovers for tomorrow)

TUESDAY

Breakfast: Breakfast burrito made with a small whole-wheat tortilla, 2 scrambled eggs, chopped tomato, and hot sauce

Lunch: Leftover Vegetable Kale Lasagna

Dinner: Roasted Beef with Peppercorn Sauce

WEDNESDAY

Breakfast: Hot oatmeal made with skim milk, topped with flaxseed and blueberries

Lunch: Creamy Mac and Cheese

Dinner: Seafood Stew

THURSDAY

Breakfast: Creamy Green Smoothie

Lunch: Wild Rice with Blueberries and Pumpkin Seeds

Dinner: Chicken tacos, made with a whole-wheat tortilla filled with shredded cooked chicken, tomatoes, lettuce, fresh cilantro, and black beans

FRIDAY

Breakfast: Spanakopita Egg White Frittata

Lunch: Mixed green salad with tomatoes, cucumber, chopped hard-boiled egg, avocado slices

Dinner: Chickpea Lentil Curry

SATURDAY

Breakfast: Lemon Blueberry Muffins

Lunch: Herbed Beans and Brown Rice

Dinner: Stir-fry with chicken or shrimp and mixed vegetables, served over brown rice

SUNDAY

Breakfast: Sweet Quinoa Cereal

Lunch: Lean turkey breast, low-fat Swiss cheese, lettuce, and tomato stuffed in a whole-wheat pita

Dinner: Spiced Lamb Stew

SNACKS

You'll notice we left the snacks out of the meal plans above. We have planned your meals so that you have enough room left for two snacks a day. In this section, you'll find a range of options for choosing snacks that fit into your diet, in terms of how many carbohydrates and calories you are eating each day. You can choose to have the snacks between breakfast and lunch, between lunch and dinner, or after dinner.

75 to 110 calories and less than 15 grams of carbohydrates

- 1 small piece of fruit (such as apple, orange, peach), and 1 ounce part-skim string cheese
- ¼ cup pomegranate seeds, and 4 ounces 0 percent or 2 percent plain Greek yogurt
- Flavored yogurt sweetened with sugar substitute, Greek or regular, light (such as Chobani Simply 100, Dannon Light & Fit Nonfat)
- ½ whole-wheat English muffin, and ⅛ avocado
- ½ ounce low-fat cheese (such as Mini Babybel light cheese), and ½ ounce whole-grain crackers (such as 2 Wasa Thin & Crispy Flatbreads)
- ½ small whole-wheat pita (½ ounce), and ½ ounce low-fat cheese spread (such as Laughing Cow)
- ½ medium apple, and 1 teaspoon almond butter
- 1 ounce nitrate-free beef or turkey jerky
- 15 large shrimp (3 ounces), and 2 tablespoons cocktail sauce
- 3 tablespoons guacamole, and 1 cup assorted raw vegetables
- 3 tablespoons hummus, and 1 cup assorted raw vegetables
- 1 small low-carb whole-wheat tortilla (such as La Tortilla Factory, Mission, Mama Lupe's), and 2 tablespoons shredded mozzarella cheese
- ½ ounce nuts (23 to 25 pistachios; 10 to 12 almonds; 2 tablespoons mixed nuts; 2 tablespoons shelled pumpkin or sunflower seeds; 20 peanuts; 3 or 4 Brazil nuts; 5 to 7 walnut halves; 8 to 9 cashew halves)

Occasional Snacks

These snacks tend to contain fewer nutrients and more added sugar than the others listed in this section, so limit them to a few times a week. Until the new food labels come out, which will differentiate added sugars from natural sugars (such as those found in fruit and yogurt), you'll just have to do your best to be a label detective. Read the ingredient list to make sure an added sugar is not one of the first ingredients. Look for products with 100 calories or less, and no more than 15 grams of carbohydrates. It should contain 8 grams of sugar or less. Some examples:

- 1 Enlightened ice cream bar
- ½ cup Breyer's No Sugar Added Vanilla Bean ice cream
- 1 So Delicious Coconutmilk Dairy-Free Frozen Dessert Fudge Bar Mini
- ½ ounce dark chocolate (such as Dove Dark Chocolate, 2 pieces)

175 to 220 calories and 30 grams of carbohydrates or less

- 1 ounce nuts (47 to 49 pistachios; 20 to 24 almonds; ¼ cup mixed nuts; ¼ cup shelled pumpkin or sunflower seeds; 40 peanuts; 6 to 8 Brazil nuts; 10 to 14 walnut halves; 16 to 18 cashew halves)
- ½ cup blueberries or 9 frozen cherries, and 6 ounces 0 percent to 2 percent plain Greek yogurt, and 1 tablespoon sunflower seeds
- 2 ounces smoked salmon, tomato slices, and 1 tablespoon low-fat cream cheese, on 2 high-fiber crackers (such as Wasa Light Rye Crispbread)
- 1 medium baked apple with cinnamon, and 7 crushed walnut halves
- ⅓ avocado, and 1 whole-wheat English muffin
- 1 medium banana, and 1 tablespoon peanut butter
- ½ cup low-fat cottage cheese, and 1 medium peach
- 15 baked tortilla chips (1 ounce), and 3 tablespoons guacamole
- ¼ cup hummus, and 1 ounce whole-grain pretzels
- Smoothie: 1 scoop low-carb protein powder or 4 ounces Greek yogurt, ¾ cup frozen berries, 4 ounces unsweetened almond milk, and 2 teaspoons ground flaxseeds

Energy Bars

Look for bars that contain 200 calories or less, with 30 grams of carbohydrates or less, and at least 5 grams of fiber. Sugar should not be one of the first ingredients. Ideally, look for a product with less than 8 grams of sugar. Some examples:

- Quest bars, such as Cookies and Cream
- Kind Dark Chocolate, Nuts and Sea Salt bar

COMMON CHALLENGES AND HOW TO DEAL WITH THEM

While diabetes is certainly a manageable disease, it can be accompanied by numerous challenges in several areas, including medical, nutritional, emotional, and social. Here are some of the more common diabetic challenges, and tips on how to deal with them.

Depression

People with diabetes have a greater risk of depression than people without diabetes. This is not surprising, considering that diabetes can be a lot to manage. People who are depressed tend to find it harder to stick with their diabetes treatment plan. Symptoms of depression include loss of energy, loss of interest in things you used to enjoy, sleeping more or less than usual, changes in appetite, feelings of guilt or worthlessness, and suicidal thoughts.

It's normal to feel sad or anxious on occasion, but if you find these thoughts are reoccurring and affecting your enjoyment of life or diabetes self-care, it is important to discuss it with your doctor. Depression can be treated with therapy and/or medication. It can also be helpful to find a local support group or online community for people with type 2 diabetes.

Hypoglycemia

While blood sugar tends to be too high if you have diabetes, certain diabetes medications and insulin can have the opposite effect, causing blood sugar to drop too low (generally under 70) at times. This is called hypoglycemia, and it can be due to eating less or exercising more than usual. Symptoms can include mental confusion, blurred vision, dizziness, feeling faint, forgetfulness, heart palpitations, mood swings, emotional outbursts, and headaches.

If this happens, you should check your blood sugar and eat about 15 grams of carbohydrate in the form of glucose tablets or 4 ounces of juice or some crackers. To prevent hypoglycemia, do your best to follow your individual diabetes treatment plan. If you experience hypoglycemia often, it's important to discuss this with your doctor, as you may need to change your treatment plan.

Feeling Overwhelmed

A major part of your treatment plan involves healthy meal planning, exercise, and stress management. But hectic schedules can make it difficult to fit all this in. When you add in a demanding job, caring for a family, and social obligations, it is no wonder if you feel exhausted and overwhelmed. What helps many of my patients is to work on small changes—which eventually add up to help with blood sugar management.

For example, set two goals for week one: walking for 20 minutes three times a week and planning meals for the week on Sunday. Week two: add in cooking dinner at home on Monday and Wednesday. As each week goes by, add in another small goal.

It can also help to ask for support. Maybe a family member can pitch in with grocery shopping, cooking, and/or cleanup. If you need help with a more detailed meal plan, make an appointment with a registered dietitian and/or certified diabetes educator. Set up an appointment with a personal trainer to get advice on an exercise routine. Meet with a therapist to get counseling for stress or depression. Getting support from others takes the load off you.

Checking Blood Sugar

You and your doctor may decide that checking your own blood sugar regularly will be part of your diabetes treatment plan. This can feel challenging and inconvenient. In addition, the blood glucose numbers can leave you feeling frustrated or angry. It is easy to do, but try not to judge yourself based on the numbers.

It is important to remind yourself that blood glucose numbers are a way of tracking how your diabetes care plan is working for you—it is not saying you are "good" or "bad." Understanding blood sugar patterns can help you achieve better control, which will ultimately decrease your risk of complications. If your numbers are consistently too high or too low, it may mean your meal plan or exercise routine needs to be revised. Or it could mean your medications need to be adjusted. If you continue to feel overwhelmed by your blood sugar testing schedule, talk to your doctor. Maybe it can be changed to better fit your needs.

SOCIAL CHALLENGES

Food is an important element of most social interactions, and this poses extra challenges for people with diabetes. Here are some ideas for how to navigate the tangled web of temptations and social pressures.

Parties and Holidays

Parties tend to revolve around food. This can be challenging if you are trying to watch your carbohydrates and your weight. The trick is to plan ahead as best as you can. If you know the host, ask what will be served. Offer to bring a healthy dish. Don't go to the party hungry. Have a light snack, ideally containing some protein, before you go. Greek yogurt or peanut butter and crackers would be a good option.

Once you get to the party, survey the foods on offer. Fill your plate up with the healthiest options. Be selective, but do not totally deprive yourself. If you really want some mac and cheese, take a small portion, but skip the rolls and potato. If you see your favorite brownies, then skip the mac and cheese and go for a small brownie. Hold a glass of club soda in your hand, and don't stand or sit near the tempting foods.

Tempting Goodies in the Office

Whether it is holiday time or a colleague's birthday, chances are that tempting goodies loaded with sugar and calories will be available. For someone with type 2 diabetes who is trying to limit their carbohydrates, this can be a tricky time. Try keeping your own healthy snacks in the office so while the others dig into the cake, you can have your apple.

If you feel close to some of your coworkers, you may want to confide in them that you have diabetes and are trying to limit your intake of sugary foods. They could end up being a good support system. If you would really like to have a small piece of birthday cake, the key word is "small." Maybe skip your afternoon snack that day. While this is not the best habit to get into, all foods can fit into a healthy diet for diabetes if you plan for them.

Happy Hour

Alcohol can fit into a healthy eating plan for people with type 2 diabetes, but there are a few things to keep in mind. Alcohol can cause low blood sugar if you are taking insulin or certain oral medications and haven't eaten, or high blood sugar if it contains a sweet

Get Your Rest

Quality sleep plays a major role in good health. Regularly getting fewer than seven hours of sleep a night can wreak havoc on blood glucose levels and insulin resistance. Insufficient sleep affects metabolic and biological processes in the body. Glucose levels rise and insulin is secreted. Leptin—the protein that tells us we've had enough food—is decreased. There is also a connection between inadequate sleep, heart disease, and obesity.

These tips to improve sleep come from the National Sleep Foundation.

♦ Stick to the same bedtime and wake time, even on the weekends.

♦ Practice a relaxing bedtime ritual. Avoid bright lights and stressful conversations. Reading is a good way to calm down.

♦ If you have trouble sleeping at night, avoid naps, especially in the afternoon.

♦ Exercise daily.

♦ Evaluate your sleep environment. Ideally, it should be cool—between 60 and 67 degrees—and free from noise or other distractions, like light. Consider using blackout curtains, eye shades, earplugs, white noise machines, humidifiers, fans, or other devices.

♦ Use bright light to help manage your circadian rhythms. Avoid bright light in the evening and expose yourself to bright light (ideally, sunlight) in the morning. This will help keep your circadian rhythms regular.

♦ Avoid alcohol, cigarettes, and heavy meals in the evening.

♦ Avoid electronics before bed or in the middle of the night, because the particular type of light emanating from the screens of these devices is activating to the brain. So if you read before bed, stick with traditional printed material.

♦ If you're still having trouble sleeping, speak with your doctor.

mixer like juice or soda. In addition, alcohol is a source of empty calories and can cause you to become less disciplined about what you eat. So moderation is the key! Stick to drinks without sweet mixers, like wine, vodka with club soda, or rum and diet cola. Try to alternate nonalcoholic drinks like club soda with the alcoholic drinks. Remember, the overall goal for health is one drink a day for women and two for men.

Food Pushers

"Come on, one little bite won't hurt you." You know the type—people who get a little pushy when they are trying to get you to eat something. Maybe giving food is how they show they care, or maybe they want you to join in so they don't feel guilty eating alone. Your best bet is to be firm and say something nice like, "Thank you. It looks delicious, but I'm not hungry right now." If they continue to push, consider telling them that you have diabetes. Often times, food pushers back off when a medical condition is mentioned.

Tempting Foods at Home

While you want to do your best to keep your kitchen diabetes-friendly, there will likely be times when other family members want to keep their favorite not-so-healthy foods around. If you find these foods difficult to stay away from, see if you can come up with a compromise. Maybe you can buy them a flavor of ice cream or potato chips that they enjoy but that does not tempt you. Keep their snacks out of sight. And make sure you have your own healthy snacks available for when your partner goes for the ice cream!

RESTAURANT DINING

Most of us don't always have time to prepare healthy meals at home and end up eating out an average of four times a week. Unfortunately, many restaurant portions are jumbo size and can wreak havoc on your blood sugar and waistline if you aren't careful. The good news is that even with diabetes, you can still have an enjoyable dining experience if you plan ahead and choose wisely. Here are some tips.

- Check out the menu ahead of time online to see if they offer healthy choices that are not fried or in a heavy sauce. Some chain restaurants even post the nutritional information of their food online.
- Don't go to the restaurant hungry. Have a light snack before you go.
- If you aren't sure how the food is prepared, ask your server. Don't assume!
- Ask to have food prepared the way you want it. If they will not accommodate you, order something else.
- If your meal comes with a starch, such as rice or potato, skip the bread. Or if you love the bread, take a piece and order extra vegetables with your meal instead of the starch.
- Ask for substitutions. Get a baked potato instead of fries or extra vegetables instead of mashed potatoes.

- Ask for a half order of pasta or split a full order with a friend.
- Avoid breaded or fried foods, or foods in heavy sauces. Look for grilled or poached fish, chicken, or lean meat.
- Get salad dressing and sauces on the side.
- Order two healthy appetizers instead of an entrée.
- Limit alcohol to one serving, and skip the fancy drinks such as margaritas.
- Try to skip dessert. But if they are serving your favorite dessert, share it with a few other people and skip the starch with your meal.
- Avoid all-you-can-eat buffets.
- Take a walk after dinner.

MINDFUL EATING

Most of us have hectic lives and tend to eat on autopilot. We make about 250 food decisions every day, and most of those decisions have nothing to do with real hunger. We eat for other reasons, including stress, boredom, social occasions, or the sight or smell of food. Mindful eating is a practice of becoming aware of your thoughts, feelings, and physical sensations as you eat. It can help you enjoy your food more, eat only when you are truly hungry, and curb your overall intake of calories. Here are some tips to get you started practicing mindful eating.

- Eat in a distraction-free environment. Turn off everything with a screen!
- Sit down. Don't eat out of the refrigerator.
- Use a smaller plate. Serve yourself one portion and put the rest away. Try not to have family-style bowls on the kitchen table.
- Pay attention to the food in front of you. Put aside thoughts of work, picking up the kids, and cleaning.
- Consider where the food came from, what it looks like on the plant or in the ground, and who grew or raised it. This creates a sense of gratitude. Appreciation for your food is a key factor in mindful eating.
- Eat slowly and savor each bite. Pay attention to how the food tastes. Put your utensils down in between bites.
- Novel ways to slow down your eating include using chopsticks or your nondominant hand.
- Pay attention to your degree of fullness. Eat only until you are satisfied, leaving yourself neither stuffed nor starving.
- Occasionally eat your meals in silence. While it is social to eat with other people, eating alone from time to time can help you focus on mindful eating—whether it is a 15-minute breakfast or a leisurely dinner.

PART TWO

The Recipes

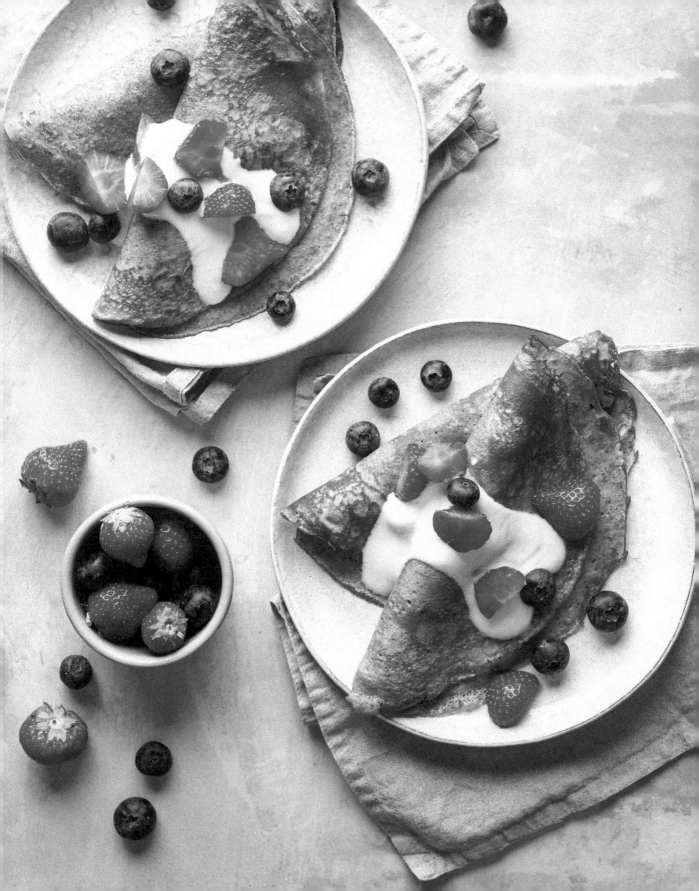

CHAPTER 4

Balanced Breakfasts

Creamy Green Smoothie

CARBS PER SERVING: 20G

SERVES 2 / PREP TIME: 5 MINUTES

Almond milk has a fresh, delicate flavor that is perfect for smoothies such as this nutritious drink. The other ingredients shine through, especially the tart green apple. Diabetes support organizations recommend nondairy or low-fat dairy milks, and almond milk has the best nutrition profile of the nondairy choices. Almond milk is cholesterol-free, low-sodium, low-calorie, and is high in vitamins A, B, D, and E.

2 cups shredded kale

½ avocado, diced

½ Granny Smith apple, unpeeled, cored and chopped

1 cup unsweetened almond milk

¼ cup 2 percent plain Greek yogurt

3 ice cubes

1. Put the kale, avocado, apple, almond milk, yogurt, and ice in a blender and blend until smooth and thick.

2. Pour into two glasses and serve.

NUTRITION TIP: *Apple skin is packed with fiber—over 50 percent of the total for this fruit—as well as containing at least 25 percent of the vitamins. The skin also contains quercetin, an antioxidant that helps protect the memory and improve breathing function.*

Per Serving Calories: 172; Total Fat: 7g; Cholesterol: 6mg; Sodium: 110mg; Total Carbohydrates: 20g; Sugar: 12g; Fiber: 4g; Protein: 8g

Oatmeal Strawberry Smoothie

CARBS PER SERVING: 27G

SERVES 2 / PREP TIME: 5 MINUTES

When you think of oatmeal, a steaming bowl of hot cereal topped with a dash of milk probably comes to mind. So whipping up oats into a pretty pink smoothie might be an unfamiliar variation. Oatmeal is an incredible addition to your morning meal because it is digested slowly and helps stabilize blood sugar. This means you will be full longer and you won't feel those frustrating midmorning cravings for sugar or carbs.

2 tablespoons instant oats
1 cup frozen strawberries
3 cups skim milk
½ teaspoon pure
    vanilla extract

1. Put the oats, strawberries, milk, and vanilla in a blender and blend until smooth.

2. Pour into two glasses and serve.

SUBSTITUTION TIP: *If you want a vegan smoothie, replace the skim milk with your favorite nut or rice milk. Always use unsweetened products to avoid added sugar, which can affect your blood sugar.*

Per Serving Calories: 166; Total Fat: 1g; Cholesterol: 5mg; Sodium: 131mg; Total Carbohydrates: 27g; Sugar: 17g; Fiber: 3g; Protein: 11g

Fruity Avocado Smoothie

CARBS PER SERVING: 25G

SERVES 2 / PREP TIME: 5 MINUTES

Traditional wisdom is not to judge a book by its cover—or in this case the smoothie by its color. Otherwise, the murky grayish hue of this smoothie could put you off drinking it. The banana and blueberries ensure the taste is sweet, and the avocado creates a luscious, creamy texture. Try whipping up a glass as a filling snack on days when you need a bit more energy.

1 cup fresh spinach
½ avocado, peeled, pitted, and diced
½ ripe banana, peeled
½ cup blueberries
2 cups unsweetened almond milk
3 ice cubes

1. Put the spinach, avocado, banana, blueberries, almond milk, and ice cubes in a blender and blend until smooth.

2. Pour into two glasses and serve.

SUBSTITUTION TIP: *Any dark leafy green will do for this sweet smoothie. Kale, beet greens, Swiss chard, or collard greens pack a similar nutrition punch, but the flavor will change slightly depending on your choice.*

Per Serving Calories: 190; Total Fat: 6g; Cholesterol: 5mg; Sodium: 144mg; Total Carbohydrates: 25g; Sugar: 17g; Fiber: 4g; Protein: 10g

Plum Smoothie

CARBS PER SERVING: 26G

SERVES 2 / PREP TIME: 5 MINUTES

Any type of plum will be delightful in this recipe, but if you have a selection of options available, sweet, juicy black plums are the best choice. Plums are very high in antioxidants, such as neochlorogenic and chlorogenic acids, which have been shown to prevent or minimize oxygen-based damage to cells. Plums can also help increase iron absorption because they are an excellent source of vitamin C.

4 ripe plums, pitted

1 cup skim milk

6 ounces 2 percent plain
   Greek yogurt

4 ice cubes

¼ teaspoon ground nutmeg

1. Put the plums, milk, yogurt, ice, and nutmeg in a blender and blend until smooth.

2. Pour into two glasses and serve.

Per Serving Calories: 157; Total Fat: 2g; Cholesterol: 8mg; Sodium: 123mg; Total Carbohydrates: 26g; Sugar: 22g; Fiber: 2g; Protein: 10g

Spicy Tomato Smoothie

CARBS PER SERVING: 12G

SERVES 2 / PREP TIME: 5 MINUTES

Smoothies are often sweet, so it can be a pleasant change to enjoy what is, in essence, gazpacho in a glass for breakfast. Try to find tomato juice with as few ingredients as possible and low salt, so the seasonings do not overwhelm the flavors of the other vegetables. If you have extra time, a topping of chopped fresh tomatoes, cucumber, and even a little jalapeño make this a guest-worthy start to the day.

1 cup tomato juice
2 tomatoes, diced
¼ English cucumber
Juice of 1 lemon
1 teaspoon hot sauce
4 ice cubes

1. Put the tomato juice, tomatoes, cucumber, lemon juice, hot sauce, and ice cubes in a blender and blend until smooth.

2. Pour into two glasses and serve.

INGREDIENT TIP: *Hot sauce covers a huge, delicious range of possibilities, from Tabasco to a secret homemade concoction featuring habanero peppers. Let your heat tolerance guide your choice, or leave the hot sauce out entirely.*

Per Serving Calories: 53; Total Fat: 0g; Cholesterol: 0mg; Sodium: 11mg; Total Carbohydrates: 12g; Sugar: 7g; Fiber: 3g; Protein: 2g

Tzatziki Smoothie

CARBS PER SERVING: 26G

SERVES 2 / PREP TIME: 5 MINUTES

Apples are the complete package—sweet, crunchy, convenient, and incredibly nutritious. Apples are essential additions to a meal plan focused on managing type 2 diabetes because they are extremely high in fiber, including a soluble fiber called pectin. Pectin helps release blood sugar into the bloodstream at a slower rate, which controls blood sugar levels in the body. Make sure you leave the skin on your apple after scrubbing it thoroughly, because the skin also contains a great deal of fiber.

2 English cucumbers, cut into chunks

1 cup 2 percent plain Greek yogurt

1 apple, unpeeled, cored and chopped

Juice of 1 lemon

3 ice cubes

1. Put the cucumbers, yogurt, apple, lemon juice, and ice cubes in a blender and blend until very smooth.

2. Pour into two glasses and serve.

Per Serving Calories: 136; Total Fat: 2g; Cholesterol: 5mg; Sodium: 65mg; Total Carbohydrates: 26g; Sugar: 18g; Fiber: 2g; Protein: 7g

Carrot Pear Smoothie

CARBS PER SERVING: 19G

SERVES 2 / PREP TIME: 10 MINUTES

Pears add a delightful sweetness and generous dose of fiber to this sunny-hued smoothie. Dietary fiber is important for managing body weight and keeping blood sugar under control. Pears are also high in copper, vitamin C, and vitamin K, which can help prevent colon and breast cancer and protect against degenerative diseases.

2 carrots, peeled and grated
1 ripe pear, unpeeled, cored and chopped
2 teaspoons grated fresh ginger
Juice and zest of 1 lime
1 cup water
½ teaspoon ground cinnamon
¼ teaspoon ground nutmeg

1. Put the carrots, pear, ginger, lime juice, lime zest, water, cinnamon, and nutmeg in a blender and blend until smooth.

2. Pour into two glasses and serve.

NUTRITION TIP: *Ginger is most often associated with improving digestive concerns, but it can also help lower fasting blood sugar levels in people with type 2 diabetes.*

Per Serving Calories: 74; Total Fat: 0g; Cholesterol: 0mg; Sodium: 43mg; Total Carbohydrates: 19g; Sugar: 11g; Fiber: 4g; Protein: 1g

Lemon Blueberry Muffins

CARBS PER SERVING: 18G

MAKES 18 MUFFINS / PREP TIME: 10 MINUTES / COOK TIME: 25 MINUTES

Muffins seem like a decadent treat, since they are like marvelous little cakes in their individual wrappers. Lemon and blueberry is a classic combination because the tartness of the citrus is perfectly balanced by the sweet plump berries. If you cannot find good fresh blueberries, you can use frozen. Add the frozen berries unthawed and with as little stirring as possible, so your muffins don't end up purple.

2 cups whole-wheat
    pastry flour
1 cup almond flour
½ cup granulated sweetener
1 tablespoon baking powder
2 teaspoons freshly grated
    lemon zest
¾ teaspoon baking soda
¾ teaspoon ground nutmeg
Pinch sea salt
2 eggs
1 cup skim milk, at
    room temperature
¾ cup 2 percent plain
    Greek yogurt
½ cup melted coconut oil
1 tablespoon freshly
    squeezed lemon juice
1 teaspoon pure
    vanilla extract
1 cup fresh blueberries

1. Preheat the oven to 350°F.

2. Line 18 muffin cups with paper liners and set the tray aside.

3. In a large bowl, stir together the flour, almond flour, sweetener, baking powder, lemon zest, baking soda, nutmeg, and salt.

4. In a small bowl, whisk together the eggs, milk, yogurt, coconut oil, lemon juice, and vanilla.

5. Add the wet ingredients to the dry ingredients and stir until just combined.

6. Fold in the blueberries without crushing them.

7. Spoon the batter evenly into the muffin cups. Bake the muffins until a toothpick inserted in the middle comes out clean, about 25 minutes.

8. Cool the muffins completely and serve.

9. Store leftover muffins in a sealed container in the refrigerator for up to 3 days or in the freezer for up to 1 month.

INGREDIENT TIP: *You can make your own almond flour by pulsing blanched whole almonds in a food processor until you get the desired texture.*

Per Serving Calories: 165; Total Fat: 9g; Cholesterol: 25mg; Sodium: 74mg; Total Carbohydrates: 18g; Sugar: 7g; Fiber: 2g; Protein: 4g

Bran Apple Muffins

CARBS PER SERVING: 19G

MAKES 18 MUFFINS / PREP TIME: 10 MINUTES / COOK TIME: 20 MINUTES

Bran muffins have a bad rep as dry and tasteless, but these lightly spiced muffins are moist with chunks of apple and flavored with vanilla. They also freeze beautifully, so put together a double batch to ensure you have a nutritious grab-and-go breakfast whenever you are running behind in the morning. You should never skip breakfast, because it can seriously affect your blood sugar.

2 cups whole-wheat flour
1 cup wheat bran
⅓ cup granulated sweetener
1 tablespoon baking powder
2 teaspoons ground cinnamon
½ teaspoon ground ginger
¼ teaspoon ground nutmeg
Pinch sea salt
2 eggs
1½ cups skim milk,
    at room temperature
½ cup melted coconut oil
2 teaspoons pure
    vanilla extract
2 apples, peeled, cored,
    and diced

1. Preheat the oven to 350°F.

2. Line 18 muffin cups with paper liners and set the tray aside.

3. In a large bowl, stir together the flour, bran, sweetener, baking powder, cinnamon, ginger, nutmeg, and salt.

4. In a small bowl, whisk the eggs, milk, coconut oil, and vanilla until blended.

5. Add the wet ingredients to the dry ingredients, stirring until just blended.

6. Stir in the apples and spoon equal amounts of batter into each muffin cup.

7. Bake the muffins until a toothpick inserted in the center of a muffin comes out clean, about 20 minutes.

8. Cool the muffins completely and serve.

9. Store leftover muffins in a sealed container in the refrigerator for up to 3 days or in the freezer for up to 1 month.

Per Serving Calories: 141; Total Fat: 7g; Cholesterol: 24mg; Sodium: 20mg; Total Carbohydrates: 19g; Sugar: 6g; Fiber: 3g; Protein: 4g

Sweet Quinoa Cereal

CARBS PER SERVING: 39G

SERVES 4 / PREP TIME: 5 MINUTES / COOK TIME: 20 MINUTES

Hot cereal gets a new look when you replace traditional oats with nutritional powerhouse quinoa. The texture is a little different, and it is important to have enough liquid left so the cereal is creamy rather than grainy. You might want to serve this quinoa cereal with a splash of skim milk or almond milk in addition to the berries and nuts.

1 cup water

1 cup skim milk

1 cup uncooked quinoa, well rinsed

½ teaspoon ground cinnamon

Pinch sea salt

2 tablespoons granulated sweetener

1 teaspoon pure vanilla extract

¼ cup toasted chopped almonds

½ cup sliced strawberries

1. Put the water, milk, quinoa, cinnamon, and salt in a medium saucepan over medium-high heat.

2. Bring the mixture to a boil, then reduce the heat to low.

3. Simmer the quinoa cereal until most of the liquid is gone, about 15 minutes.

4. Remove the cereal from the heat and stir in the sweetener and vanilla.

5. Spoon the cereal into four bowls and top with the almonds and strawberries.

NUTRITION TIP: *If you are looking for disease-busting phytonutrients and antioxidants, look no further than quinoa. This pseudo-cereal contains quercetin, kaempferol, coumaric, and omega-3 fatty acids, as well as a generous amount of fiber.*

Per Serving Calories: 259; Total Fat: 7g; Cholesterol: 1mg; Sodium: 38mg; Total Carbohydrates: 39g; Sugar: 10g; Fiber: 4g; Protein: 10g

Simple Buckwheat Porridge

CARBS PER SERVING: 22G

SERVES 4 / PREP TIME: 5 MINUTES / COOK TIME: 40 MINUTES

Porridge sounds quaintly old-fashioned and wholesome, like you would be eating it in a cabin in the middle of a pristine forest before doing chores. Porridge is really just a starchy plant—usually grain—crushed and boiled in water or another liquid such as milk. Buckwheat porridge is often served in Russia and the Ukraine with a generous dollop of butter or yogurt, which can be added just before you enjoy this filling breakfast.

2 cups raw buckwheat groats
3 cups water
Pinch sea salt
1 cup unsweetened
   almond milk

1. Put the buckwheat groats, water, and salt in a medium saucepan over medium-high heat.

2. Bring the mixture to a boil, then reduce the heat to low.

3. Cook until most of the water is absorbed, about 20 minutes. Stir in the milk and cook until very soft, about 15 minutes.

4. Serve the porridge with your favorite toppings such as chopped nuts, sliced banana, or fresh berries.

INGREDIENT TIP: *Buckwheat can be found in most grocery stores in the bulk section or the organic/health food section. Buckwheat is actually a seed that is gluten-free and a stellar source of fiber.*

Per Serving Calories: 122; Total Fat: 1g; Cholesterol: 1mg; Sodium: 48mg; Total Carbohydrates: 22g; Sugar: 4g; Fiber: 3g; Protein: 6g

Easy Breakfast Chia Pudding

CARBS PER SERVING: 25G

SERVES 4 / PREP TIME: 5 MINUTES, PLUS 1 HOUR CHILLING TIME

Chia seeds seem a bit like a science project when you see how much liquid these little seeds absorb to create a thick pudding: about 12 times their weight. This spectacular absorption rate is important, because the gel-like consistency will slow digestion and decrease sugar spikes. Soaked chia seeds also decrease cholesterol and support healthy bones and teeth. Chia seeds are an excellent source of protein, fiber, manganese, phosphorus, calcium, and omega-3 fatty acids.

4 cups unsweetened almond milk or skim milk
¾ cup chia seeds
1 teaspoon ground cinnamon
Pinch sea salt

1. Stir together the milk, chia seeds, cinnamon, and salt in a medium bowl.

2. Cover the bowl with plastic wrap and chill in the refrigerator until the pudding is thick, about 1 hour.

3. Sweeten with your favorite sweetener and fruit.

Per Serving Calories: 237; Total Fat: 10g; Cholesterol: 5mg; Sodium: 134mg; Total Carbohydrates: 25g; Sugar: 12g; Fiber: 11g; Protein: 13g

Baked Berry Coconut Oatmeal

CARBS PER SERVING: 27G

SERVES 6 / PREP TIME: 10 MINUTES / COOK TIME: 35 MINUTES

Sometimes cooking oatmeal from scratch can result in a thick, gelatinous mess because you cook it too fast, or add too many oats or too little liquid. Baked oatmeal eliminates that frustration by taking the guesswork out of breakfast, and you don't have to spend time stirring the cereal over a hot stove.

2 cups rolled oats
¼ cup shredded
    unsweetened coconut
1 teaspoon baking powder
½ teaspoon ground cinnamon
¼ teaspoon sea salt
2 cups skim milk
¼ cup melted coconut oil,
    plus extra for greasing the
    baking dish
1 egg
1 teaspoon pure
    vanilla extract
2 cups fresh blueberries
⅛ cup chopped pecans,
    for garnish
1 teaspoon chopped fresh
    mint leaves, for garnish

1. Preheat the oven to 350°F.

2. Lightly oil a 2-quart baking dish and set it aside.

3. In a medium bowl, stir together the oats, coconut, baking powder, cinnamon, and salt.

4. In a small bowl, whisk together the milk, oil, egg, and vanilla until well blended.

5. Layer half the dry ingredients in the baking dish, top with half the berries, then spoon the remaining half of the dry ingredients and the rest of the berries on top.

6. Pour the wet ingredients evenly into the baking dish. Tap it lightly on the counter to disperse the wet ingredients throughout.

7. Bake the casserole, uncovered, until the oats are tender, about 35 minutes.

8. Serve immediately, topped with the pecans and mint.

COOKING TIP: *The best part about serving a casserole is that you can assemble it the evening before, and then pop it in the oven with no mess or fuss in the morning.*

Per Serving Calories: 295; Total Fat: 17g; Cholesterol: 37mg; Sodium: 154mg; Total Carbohydrates: 27g; Sugar: 11g; Fiber: 4g; Protein: 10g

Vanilla Steel-Cut Oatmeal

CARBS PER SERVING: 30G

SERVES 4 / PREP TIME: 5 MINUTES / COOK TIME: 40 MINUTES

Vanilla is a popular flavor that can be intensified by using a vanilla bean instead of extract. You still get all the delightful taste of extract, but more health benefits come from the bean. Vanilla beans contain B vitamins, zinc, calcium, iron, and potassium. This means vanilla beans are heart-friendly and bone-friendly. If you want to try using a bean in this recipe, cut one in half lengthwise and scrape the seeds into the water before bringing it to a boil.

4 cups water
Pinch sea salt
1 cup steel-cut oats
¾ cup skim milk
2 teaspoons pure
vanilla extract

1. In a large pot over high heat, bring the water and salt to a boil.

2. Reduce the heat to low and stir in the oats.

3. Cook the oats for about 30 minutes to soften, stirring occasionally.

4. Stir in the milk and vanilla and cook until your desired consistency is reached, about 10 more minutes.

5. Remove the cereal from the heat. Serve topped with sunflower seeds, chopped peaches, fresh berries, sliced almonds, or flaxseeds.

Per Serving Calories: 186; Total Fat: 0g; Cholesterol: 1mg; Sodium: 36mg; Total Carbohydrates: 30g; Sugar: 2g; Fiber: 5g; Protein: 9g

Spanakopita Egg White Frittata

CARBS PER SERVING: 4G

SERVES 4 / PREP TIME: 10 MINUTES / COOK TIME: 15 MINUTES

Spinach and feta cheese packed into savory little pockets for cocktail parties is probably where you have seen spanakopita in the past. This combination also works well for a pretty baked frittata. You can blanch the spinach before adding it to the eggs if you want a creamier texture, but make sure you squeeze out all the water from the cooked greens to avoid sogginess.

2 tablespoons extra-virgin olive oil

½ sweet onion, chopped

1 red bell pepper, seeded and chopped

½ teaspoon minced garlic

¼ teaspoon sea salt

½ teaspoon freshly ground black pepper

8 egg whites

2 cups shredded spinach

½ cup crumbled low-sodium feta cheese

1 teaspoon chopped fresh parsley, for garnish

1. Preheat the oven to 375°F.

2. Place a heavy ovenproof skillet over medium-high heat and add the olive oil.

3. Sauté the onion, bell pepper, and garlic until softened, about 5 minutes. Season with salt and pepper.

4. Whisk together the egg whites in a medium bowl, then pour them into the skillet and lightly shake the pan to disburse.

5. Cook the vegetables and eggs for 3 minutes, without stirring.

6. Scatter the spinach over the eggs and sprinkle the feta cheese evenly over the spinach.

7. Put the skillet in the oven and bake, uncovered, until cooked through and firm, about 10 minutes.

8. Loosen the edges of the frittata with a rubber spatula, then invert it onto a plate.

9. Garnish with the chopped parsley and serve.

SUBSTITUTION TIP: *Whole eggs can be used instead of whites, substituting 6 eggs for the 8 whites. Whole eggs will increase the calories, fat, and cholesterol in the finished dish.*

Per Serving Calories: 145; Total Fat: 10g; Cholesterol: 12mg; Sodium: 291mg; Total Carbohydrates: 4g; Sugar: 3g; Fiber: 1g; Protein: 10g

Broccoli Cheese Breakfast Casserole

CARBS PER SERVING: 5G

SERVES 4 / PREP TIME: 10 MINUTES / COOK TIME: 40 MINUTES

Broccoli is one of the loveliest vegetables you will ever cut up, with its vibrant green color and tightly packed florets. This cruciferous vegetable can lower cholesterol due to its ability to bind bile acids, thereby helping the body excrete those acids. Broccoli is an effective detoxifier, fights cancer, and boosts the immune system. Look for florets with firm stalks and no yellowing or wet spots.

2 tablespoons extra-virgin olive oil
1 cup sliced button mushrooms
½ sweet onion, chopped
1 teaspoon minced garlic
1 cup chopped broccoli
8 large eggs
¼ cup skim milk
1 tablespoon chopped fresh basil
1 cup shredded fat-free Cheddar cheese
Sea salt
Freshly ground black pepper

1. Preheat the oven to 375°F.

2. Place a large ovenproof skillet over medium-high heat and add the olive oil.

3. Sauté the mushrooms, onion, and garlic until tender, about 5 minutes.

4. Add the broccoli and sauté for 5 minutes.

5. In a small bowl, whisk together the eggs, milk, and basil.

6. Remove the skillet from the heat and pour the egg mixture evenly over the vegetables.

7. Sprinkle the cheese over the casserole and bake, uncovered, until the eggs are puffy, about 30 minutes.

8. Season with salt and pepper. Serve hot or cold.

Per Serving Calories: 273; Total Fat: 19g; Cholesterol: 429mg; Sodium: 342mg; Total Carbohydrates: 5g; Sugar: 3g; Fiber: 1g; Protein: 21g

Egg-Stuffed Tomatoes

CARBS PER SERVING: 10G

SERVINGS 4 / PREP TIME: 20 MINUTES, PLUS 30 MINUTES TO DRAIN /
COOK TIME: 15 MINUTES

This dish delights children because the eggs look like they are trying to hide in the tomatoes under a camouflage of tasty Swiss cheese. If the picky eaters at home do not like their eggs sunny-side up, you can certainly scramble them and simply spoon the uncooked scramble into the tomatoes instead. Be careful when measuring out the eggs, because when scrambled, they have a tendency to pour out very quickly, which could easily overflow the tomatoes.

1 teaspoon extra-virgin
    olive oil
4 large tomatoes
¼ teaspoon sea salt, plus
    more for seasoning
1 cup shredded kale
2 tablespoons heavy
    (whipping) cream
¼ cup shredded low-fat
    Swiss cheese
4 large eggs
1 tablespoon chopped
    fresh parsley
Freshly ground black pepper

1. Preheat the oven to 375°F.

2. Lightly grease an 8-by-8-inch baking dish with the olive oil and set it aside.

3. Cut the tops off the tomatoes and carefully scoop out the insides, leaving the outer shells intact.

4. Sprinkle the insides of the tomatoes with ¼ teaspoon of salt and set them cut-side down on paper towels for 30 minutes.

5. Place the tomatoes in the baking dish, hollow-side up, and evenly divide the kale between them.

6. Divide the cream and cheese between the tomatoes. Carefully crack an egg on top of the cheese in each tomato.

7. Bake the tomatoes until the eggs are set, about 15 minutes.

8. Serve the stuffed tomatoes topped with parsley and seasoned lightly with salt and pepper.

Per Serving Calories: 161; Total Fat: 10g; Cholesterol: 223mg; Sodium: 145mg; Total Carbohydrates: 10g; Sugar: 5g; Fiber: 3g; Protein: 10g

Summer Veggie Scramble

CARBS PER SERVING: 4G

SERVES 4 / PREP TIME: 10 MINUTES / COOK TIME: 10 MINUTES

The idea behind this dish is to get as many different colors into the scrambled eggs as possible, because it looks superb and because each color represents a different array of nutrients. One of the ways to ensure you eat a balanced, complete diet is to include a wide variety of colorful vegetables and fruits in your meals every day. So you can change the ingredients here, but try to stay away from a monochromatic palette.

1 teaspoon extra-virgin olive oil
1 scallion, white and green parts, finely chopped
½ yellow bell pepper, seeded and chopped
½ zucchini, diced
8 large eggs, beaten
1 tomato, cored, seeded, and diced
2 teaspoons chopped fresh oregano
Sea salt
Freshly ground black pepper

1. Place a large skillet over medium heat and add the olive oil.

2. Add the scallion, bell pepper, and zucchini to the skillet and sauté for about 5 minutes.

3. Pour in the eggs and, using a wooden spoon or spatula, scramble them until thick, firm curds form and the eggs are cooked through, about 5 minutes.

4. Add the tomato and oregano to the skillet and stir to incorporate.

5. Serve seasoned with salt and pepper.

Per Serving Calories: 196; Total Fat: 11g; Cholesterol: 432mg; Sodium: 156mg; Total Carbohydrates: 4g; Sugar: 2g; Fiber: 1g; Protein: 13g

Ratatouille Baked Eggs

CARBS PER SERVING: 13G

SERVES 4 / PREP TIME: 20 MINUTES / COOK TIME: 50 MINUTES

Eggs can be cooked just about any way—except perhaps barbecued, because the eggs would just drip through the grill. Baking eggs in a fragrant vegetable stew adds another layer of flavor to the eggs, as they soak up the herbs and tomato essence as they cook. This dish would be perfectly acceptable for a hearty lunch or light dinner, as well as a leisurely breakfast.

2 teaspoons extra-virgin olive oil
½ sweet onion, finely chopped
2 teaspoons minced garlic
½ small eggplant, peeled and diced
1 green zucchini, diced
1 yellow zucchini, diced
1 red bell pepper, seeded and diced
3 tomatoes, seeded and chopped
1 tablespoon chopped fresh oregano
1 tablespoon chopped fresh basil
Pinch red pepper flakes
Sea salt
Freshly ground black pepper
4 large eggs

1. Preheat the oven to 350°F.

2. Place a large ovenproof skillet over medium heat and add the olive oil.

3. Sauté the onion and garlic until softened and translucent, about 3 minutes. Stir in the eggplant and sauté for about 10 minutes, stirring occasionally. Stir in the zucchini and pepper and sauté for 5 minutes.

4. Reduce the heat to low and cover. Cook until the vegetables are soft, about 15 minutes.

5. Stir in the tomatoes, oregano, basil, and red pepper flakes, and cook 10 minutes more. Season the ratatouille with salt and pepper.

6. Use a spoon to create four wells in the mixture. Crack an egg into each well.

7. Place the skillet in the oven and bake until the eggs are firm, about 5 minutes.

8. Remove from the oven. Serve the eggs with a generous scoop of vegetables.

COOKING TIP: *The ratatouille can be made ahead and kept in the fridge until you want to prepare your breakfast. Reheat the ratatouille in a skillet on the stove top until it's piping hot, then bake the eggs in the mixture.*

Per Serving Calories: 147; Total Fat: 8g; Cholesterol: 211mg; Sodium: 98mg; Total Carbohydrates: 13g; Sugar: 7g; Fiber: 4g; Protein: 9g

Cottage Cheese Almond Pancakes

CARBS PER SERVING: 11G

SERVES 4 / PREP TIME: 10 MINUTES / COOK TIME: 20 MINUTES

If you have ever made pancakes from scratch, you might be surprised by how fluffy and golden these cheese-based beauties turn out. Cottage cheese is made from milk curds—milk proteins that have clumped together—and has a mild, slightly tangy flavor. This product is high in protein, phosphorus, selenium, calcium, and B vitamins. Cottage cheese is often part of a weight-loss or health-related diet because it is low in calories, but the protein helps make you feel full.

2 cups low-fat cottage cheese
4 egg whites
2 eggs
1 tablespoon pure
    vanilla extract
1½ cups almond flour
Nonstick cooking spray

1. Place the cottage cheese, egg whites, eggs, and vanilla in a blender and pulse to combine.

2. Add the almond flour to the blender and blend until smooth.

3. Place a large nonstick skillet over medium heat and lightly coat it with cooking spray.

4. Spoon ¼ cup of batter per pancake, 4 at a time, into the skillet. Cook the pancakes until the bottoms are firm and golden, about 4 minutes.

5. Flip the pancakes over and cook the other side until they are cooked through, about 3 minutes.

6. Remove the pancakes to a plate and repeat with the remaining batter.

7. Serve with fresh fruit.

Per Serving Calories: 344; Total Fat: 22g; Cholesterol: 110mg; Sodium: 559mg; Total Carbohydrates: 11g; Sugar: 5g; Fiber: 4g; Protein: 29g

Greek Yogurt Cinnamon Pancakes

CARBS PER SERVING: 28G

SERVES 4 / PREP TIME: 5 MINUTES / COOK TIME: 20 MINUTES

Greek yogurt has more carbs than regular yogurt, but it has less sugar and more protein. It's also very high in immune system–boosting probiotics as well as calcium, which supports bone health. Greek yogurt is a fabulous source of potassium, B vitamins, iodine, and amino acids, too. Make sure the yogurt you buy is true strained Greek yogurt, rather than a regular product with added thickening agents and whey protein concentrate.

1 cup 2 percent plain
   Greek yogurt
3 eggs
1½ teaspoons pure
   vanilla extract
1 cup rolled oats
1 tablespoon
   granulated sweetener
1 teaspoon baking powder
1 teaspoon ground cinnamon
Pinch ground cloves
Nonstick cooking spray

1. Place the yogurt, eggs, and vanilla in a blender and pulse to combine.

2. Add the oats, sweetener, baking powder, cinnamon, and cloves to the blender and blend until the batter is smooth.

3. Place a large nonstick skillet over medium heat and lightly coat it with cooking spray.

4. Spoon ¼ cup of batter per pancake, 4 at a time, into the skillet. Cook the pancakes until the bottoms are firm and golden, about 4 minutes.

5. Flip the pancakes over and cook the other side until they are cooked through, about 3 minutes.

6. Remove the pancakes to a plate and repeat with the remaining batter.

7. Serve with fresh fruit.

Per Serving Calories: 243; Total Fat: 8g; Cholesterol: 169mg; Sodium: 81mg; Total Carbohydrates: 28g; Sugar: 3g; Fiber: 4g; Protein: 13g

Pumpkin Apple Waffles

CARBS PER SERVING: 40G

SERVES 6 / PREP TIME 10 MINUTES / COOK TIME: 20 MINUTES

The cinnamon and pumpkin scent of these autumn-themed waffles will call people to the kitchen for breakfast. There is something comforting about pumpkin; it seems to evoke memories of family gatherings during the holidays. Make sure you get pure packed pumpkin if you're using canned, because pumpkin pie filling is full of extra sugar, preservatives, and spices.

2¼ cups whole-wheat pastry flour

2 tablespoons granulated sweetener

1 tablespoon baking powder

1 teaspoon ground cinnamon

1 teaspoon ground nutmeg

4 eggs

1¼ cups pure pumpkin purée

1 apple, peeled, cored, and finely chopped

Melted coconut oil, for cooking

1. In a large bowl, stir together the flour, sweetener, baking powder, cinnamon, and nutmeg.

2. In a small bowl, whisk together the eggs and pumpkin.

3. Add the wet ingredients to the dry and whisk until smooth.

4. Stir the apple into the batter.

5. Cook the waffles according to the waffle maker manufacturer's directions, brushing your waffle iron with melted coconut oil, until all the batter is gone.

6. Serve.

COOKING TIP: *If you do not have a waffle maker, this batter is also perfectly fine for pancakes. Just spoon out about ¼ cup per pancake and cook in a nice hot skillet.*

Per Serving Calories: 231; Total Fat: 4g; Cholesterol: 141mg; Sodium: 51mg; Total Carbohydrates: 40g; Sugar: 5g; Fiber: 7g; Protein: 11g

Buckwheat Crêpes with Fruit and Yogurt

CARBS PER SERVING: 54G

SERVES 5 / PREP TIME: 20 MINUTES, PLUS 2 HOURS TO REST /
COOK TIME: 20 MINUTES

Buckwheat is a very effective choice for stabilizing blood sugar and is good for the cardiovascular system because of its magnesium content. The flavor of this grain is slightly stronger than whole-wheat or other flours, but absolutely delicious, especially when topped with bright berries and creamy yogurt. Leftover crêpes can be layered between sheets of baking parchment or wax paper, placed in resealable plastic bags, and frozen for up to 3 months.

1½ cups skim milk
3 eggs
1 teaspoon extra-virgin olive oil, plus more for the skillet
1 cup buckwheat flour
½ cup whole-wheat flour
½ cup 2 percent plain Greek yogurt
1 cup sliced strawberries
1 cup blueberries

1. In a large bowl, whisk together the milk, eggs, and 1 teaspoon of oil until well combined.

2. Into a medium bowl, sift together the buckwheat and whole-wheat flours. Add the dry ingredients to the wet ingredients and whisk until well combined and very smooth.

3. Allow the batter to rest for at least 2 hours before cooking.

4. Place a large skillet or crêpe pan over medium-high heat and lightly coat the bottom with oil.

5. Pour about ¼ cup of batter into the skillet. Swirl the pan until the batter completely coats the bottom.

6. Cook the crêpe for about 1 minute, then flip it over. Cook the other side of the crêpe for another minute, until lightly browned. Transfer the cooked crêpe to a plate and cover with a clean dish towel to keep warm.

7. Repeat until the batter is used up; you should have about 10 crêpes.

8. Spoon 1 tablespoon of yogurt onto each crêpe and place two crêpes on each plate.

9. Top with berries and serve.

Per Serving (2 crêpes) Calories: 329; Total Fat: 7g; Cholesterol: 130mg; Sodium: 102mg; Total Carbohydrates: 54g; Sugar: 11g; Fiber: 8g; Protein: 16g

Golden Potato Cakes

CARBS PER SERVING: 18G

SERVES 4 / PREP TIME: 10 MINUTES / COOK TIME: 25 MINUTES

You might be familiar with latkes, hash browns, tattie fish, rårakor, or other names for what is essentially shredded potatoes fried golden brown. Potato cakes can be found all over the world, accented by many ingredients such as onion, garlic, and eggs, and topped with apples, meats, sour cream, and even caviar, depending on the geography.

½ pound russet potatoes, peeled, shredded, rinsed, and patted dry
¼ sweet onion, chopped
1 teaspoon extra-virgin olive oil
1 teaspoon chopped fresh thyme
Sea salt
Freshly ground black pepper
Nonstick cooking spray
1 cup unsweetened applesauce

1. Place the potatoes, onion, oil, and thyme in a large bowl and stir to mix well.

2. Season the potato mixture generously with salt and pepper.

3. Place a large skillet over medium heat and lightly coat it with cooking spray.

4. Scoop about ¼ cup of potato mixture per cake into the skillet and press down with a spatula, about 4 cakes per batch.

5. Cook until the bottoms are golden brown and firm, about 5 to 7 minutes, then flip the cake over. Cook the other side until it is golden brown and the cake is completely cooked through, about 5 minutes more.

6. Remove the cakes to a plate and repeat with the remaining mixture.

7. Serve with the applesauce.

Per Serving Calories: 106; Total Fat: 3g; Cholesterol: 0mg; Sodium: 6mg; Total Carbohydrates: 18g; Sugar: 7g; Fiber: 2g; Protein: 1g

Wild Mushroom Frittata

CARBS PER SERVING: 5G

SERVES 4 / PREP TIME: 10 MINUTES / COOK TIME: 15 MINUTES

Wild mushrooms are not as hard to find as you might think, and you do not have to forage in the forest and fields to create your breakfast. Most supermarkets carry a magnificent array of fungi, from oyster to portobello and enoki. All have different textures and flavors, so get at least three types and experiment for the best possible taste. This frittata is also delicious cold, wrapped in a whole-grain tortilla, so any leftovers will be eaten quickly the next day.

8 large eggs
½ cup skim milk
¼ teaspoon ground nutmeg
Sea salt
Freshly ground black pepper
2 teaspoons extra-virgin
    olive oil
2 cups sliced wild mushrooms
    (cremini, oyster, shiitake,
    portobello, etc.)
½ red onion, chopped
1 teaspoon minced garlic
½ cup goat cheese, crumbled

1. Preheat the broiler.

2. In a medium bowl, whisk together the eggs, milk, and nutmeg until well combined. Season the egg mixture lightly with salt and pepper and set it aside.

3. Place an ovenproof skillet over medium heat and add the oil, coating the bottom completely by tilting the pan.

4. Sauté the mushrooms, onion, and garlic until translucent, about 7 minutes.

5. Pour the egg mixture into the skillet and cook until the bottom of the frittata is set, lifting the edges of the cooked egg to allow the uncooked egg to seep under.

6. Place the skillet under the broiler until the top is set, about 1 minute.

7. Sprinkle the goat cheese on the frittata and broil until the cheese is melted, about 1 minute more.

8. Remove from the oven. Cut into 4 wedges to serve.

INGREDIENT TIP: *Goat cheese used to be a specialty item only found in fine restaurants and gourmet groceries. This tangy cheese can now be found in most supermarkets next to the other cheeses. For a real treat, get your goat cheese right from the producer by visiting a farmers' market.*

Per Serving Calories: 226; Total Fat: 15g; Cholesterol: 430mg; Sodium: 223mg; Total Carbohydrates: 5g; Sugar: 4g; Fiber: 1g; Protein: 17g

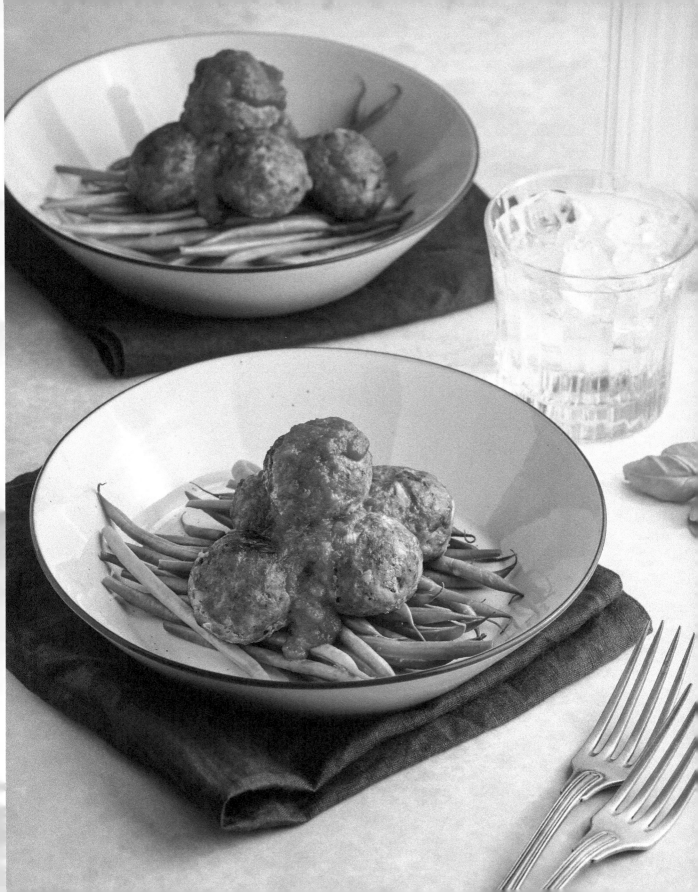

CHAPTER 5

Poultry Mains

Chicken and Roasted Vegetable Wraps

CARBS PER SERVING: 45G

SERVES 4 / PREP TIME: 10 MINUTES / COOK TIME: 20 MINUTES

Wraps are a fun way to eat an assortment of healthy ingredients, and they're useful when you're on the run, when a sandwich might be too bulky or messy. This combination of fillings would benefit from a teaspoon of chopped fresh basil or sun-dried tomato pesto spread on the tortilla. You can also toss the veggies with pesto before roasting them, for a more intense flavor. Look for lower-carb tortillas so you can easily stick to your diet plan.

½ small eggplant, cut into ¼-inch-thick slices

1 red bell pepper, seeded and cut into 1-inch-wide strips

1 medium zucchini, cut lengthwise into strips

½ small red onion, sliced

1 tablespoon extra-virgin olive oil

Sea salt

Freshly ground black pepper

2 (8-ounce) cooked chicken breasts, sliced

4 whole-wheat tortilla wraps

1. Preheat the oven to 400°F.

2. Line a baking sheet with aluminum foil and set it aside.

3. In a large bowl, toss the eggplant, bell pepper, zucchini, and red onion with the olive oil.

4. Transfer the vegetables to the baking sheet and lightly season with salt and pepper.

5. Roast the vegetables until soft and slightly charred, about 20 minutes.

6. Divide the vegetables and chicken into four portions.

7. Wrap 1 tortilla around each portion of chicken and grilled vegetables, and serve.

COOKING TIP: *Cooked chicken breasts are very handy for sandwiches, soups, and other recipes, so it makes sense to roast several at the beginning of the week. The breasts will keep for 3 to 4 days in the fridge, after you cool them completely.*

Per Serving Calories: 483; Total Fat: 25g; Cholesterol: 46mg; Sodium: 730mg; Total Carbohydrates: 45g; Sugar: 4g; Fiber: 3g; Protein: 20g

Spicy Chicken Cacciatore

CARBS PER SERVING: 14G

SERVES 6 / PREP TIME: 20 MINUTES / COOK TIME: 1 HOUR

Buying a whole chicken and cutting it up is better value, cost-wise, and the process is not difficult. You just have to use the natural contours of the bird as a guide. So, for example, cut the legs through their joints, and follow the line of bones to remove the breasts. The nutrition data for this recipe includes the skin, because it adds richness to the finished dish. You can discard it before eating your own portion.

1 (2-pound) chicken
¼ cup all-purpose flour
Sea salt
Freshly ground black pepper
2 tablespoons extra-virgin
    olive oil
3 slices bacon, chopped
1 sweet onion, chopped
2 teaspoons minced garlic
4 ounces button
    mushrooms, halved
1 (28-ounce) can low-sodium
    stewed tomatoes
½ cup red wine
2 teaspoons chopped
    fresh oregano
Pinch red pepper flakes

1. Cut the chicken into pieces: 2 drumsticks, 2 thighs, 2 wings, and 4 breast pieces.

2. Dredge the chicken pieces in the flour and season each piece with salt and pepper.

3. Place a large skillet over medium-high heat and add the olive oil.

4. Brown the chicken pieces on all sides, about 20 minutes in total. Transfer the chicken to a plate.

5. Add the chopped bacon to the skillet and cook until crispy, about 5 minutes. With a slotted spoon, transfer the cooked bacon to the same plate as the chicken.

6. Pour off most of the oil from the skillet, leaving just a light coating. Sauté the onion, garlic, and mushrooms in the skillet until tender, about 4 minutes.

7. Stir in the tomatoes, wine, oregano, and red pepper flakes.

8. Bring the sauce to a boil. Return the chicken and bacon, plus any accumulated juices from the plate, to the skillet.

9. Reduce the heat to low and simmer until the chicken is tender, about 30 minutes.

Per Serving Calories: 230; Total Fat: 17g; Cholesterol: 25mg; Sodium: 420mg; Total Carbohydrates: 14g; Sugar: 5g; Fiber: 2g; Protein: 8g

Ginger Citrus Chicken Thighs

CARBS PER SERVING: 9G

SERVES 4 / PREP TIME: 15 MINUTES / COOK TIME: 30 MINUTES

Lemons add a satisfying, fresh tartness to this ginger sauce. They have many health benefits too. They are used for detoxing, cooling heartburn, and improving conditions associated with high uric acid, such as gout. Lemons are very high in vitamin C and are recommended by the American Diabetes Association because their soluble fiber content can help stabilize blood sugar.

4 chicken thighs,
    bone-in, skinless
1 tablespoon grated
    fresh ginger
Sea salt
1 tablespoon extra-virgin
    olive oil
Juice and zest of ½ lemon
Juice and zest of ½ orange
2 tablespoons honey
1 tablespoon reduced-sodium
    soy sauce
Pinch red pepper flakes
1 tablespoon chopped
    fresh cilantro

1. Rub the chicken thighs with the ginger and season lightly with salt.

2. Place a large skillet over medium-high heat and add the oil.

3. Brown the chicken thighs, turning once, for about 10 minutes.

4. While the chicken is browning, stir together the lemon juice and zest, orange juice and zest, honey, soy sauce, and red pepper flakes in a small bowl.

5. Add the citrus mixture to the skillet, cover, and reduce the heat to low.

6. Braise until the chicken is cooked through, about 20 minutes, adding a couple of tablespoons of water if the pan is too dry.

7. Serve garnished with the cilantro.

Per Serving Calories: 114; Total Fat: 5g; Cholesterol: 34mg; Sodium: 287mg; Total Carbohydrates: 9g; Sugar: 9g; Fiber: 0g; Protein: 9g

Chicken with Creamy Thyme Sauce

CARBS PER SERVING: 4G

SERVES 4 / PREP TIME: 15 MINUTES / COOK TIME: 30 MINUTES

This is an elegant dinner party meal, and less work than you think it might take to make such a luscious sauce. Thyme is a versatile herb often found in sauces, stews, egg dishes, and sometimes even in ice cream. It is a good source of antioxidants and is traditionally considered a remedy for respiratory problems such as coughs and congestion. Thyme is also high in manganese, iron, vitamin A, fiber, and copper.

4 (4-ounce) boneless, skinless chicken breasts
Sea salt
Freshly ground black pepper
1 tablespoon extra-virgin olive oil
½ sweet onion, chopped
1 cup low-sodium chicken broth
2 teaspoons chopped fresh thyme
¼ cup heavy (whipping) cream
1 tablespoon butter
1 scallion, white and green parts, chopped

1. Preheat the oven to 375°F.

2. Season the chicken breasts lightly with salt and pepper.

3. Place a large ovenproof skillet over medium-high heat and add the olive oil.

4. Brown the chicken, turning once, about 10 minutes in total. Transfer the chicken to a plate.

5. In the same skillet, sauté the onion until softened and translucent, about 3 minutes.

6. Add the chicken broth and thyme, and simmer until the liquid has reduced by half, about 6 minutes.

7. Stir in the cream and butter, and return the chicken and any accumulated juices from the plate to the skillet.

8. Transfer the skillet to the oven. Bake until cooked through, about 10 minutes.

9. Serve topped with the chopped scallion.

Per Serving Calories: 287; Total Fat: 14g; Cholesterol: 111mg; Sodium: 184mg; Total Carbohydrates: 4g; Sugar: 1g; Fiber: 1g; Protein: 34g

One-Pot Roast Chicken Dinner

CARBS PER SERVING: 14G

SERVES 6 / PREP TIME: 10 MINUTES / COOK TIME: 40 MINUTES

One-pot meals are popular with anyone whose schedule is bursting with obligations, because you can serve a healthy dinner and still have enough time to get everything else done. The vegetables cook in the chicken juices and caramelize on the edges that are pressed against the roasting pan, giving them a complex, slightly sweet flavor. You can stir the vegetables in the middle of the cooking time so that more edges get brown and crispy.

½ head cabbage, cut into 2-inch chunks

1 sweet onion, peeled and cut into eighths

1 sweet potato, peeled and cut into 1-inch chunks

4 garlic cloves, peeled and lightly crushed

2 tablespoons extra-virgin olive oil, divided

2 teaspoons minced fresh thyme

Sea salt

Freshly ground black pepper

2½ pounds bone-in chicken thighs and drumsticks

1. Preheat the oven to 450°F.

2. Lightly grease a large roasting pan and arrange the cabbage, onion, sweet potato, and garlic in the bottom. Drizzle with 1 tablespoon of oil, sprinkle with the thyme, and season the vegetables lightly with salt and pepper.

3. Season the chicken with salt and pepper.

4. Place a large skillet over medium-high heat and brown the chicken on both sides in the remaining 1 tablespoon of oil, about 10 minutes in total.

5. Place the browned chicken on top of the vegetables in the roasting pan. Roast until the chicken is cooked through, about 30 minutes.

NUTRITION TIP: *Cabbage is a member of the cruciferous vegetable family, which are considered one of the types of vegetable you should eat every day. Cabbage can help lower cholesterol, fight against cancer, and support a healthy cardiovascular system.*

Per Serving Calories: 540; Total Fat: 34g; Cholesterol: 186mg; Sodium: 212mg; Total Carbohydrates: 14g; Sugar: 5g; Fiber: 4g; Protein: 43g

Tantalizing Jerked Chicken

CARBS PER SERVING: 3G

SERVES 4 / PREP TIME: 10 MINUTES, PLUS 4 HOURS TO MARINATE /
COOK TIME: 20 MINUTES

The spice combination used for this signature Jamaican dish varies, depending on who is doing the cooking. This version is low in sodium and relies heavily on chile peppers and a generous scoop of allspice. You can drop the heat by using a milder chile pepper, such as jalapeño, instead of the fiery habanero. Try cooking the marinated chicken on the grill for a more authentic flavor.

4 (5-ounce) boneless, skinless chicken breasts
½ sweet onion, cut into chunks
2 habanero chile peppers, halved lengthwise, seeded
¼ cup freshly squeezed lime juice
2 tablespoons extra-virgin olive oil
1 tablespoon minced garlic
1 tablespoon ground allspice
2 teaspoons chopped fresh thyme
1 teaspoon freshly ground black pepper
½ teaspoon ground nutmeg
¼ teaspoon ground cinnamon
2 cups fresh greens (such as arugula or spinach)
1 cup halved cherry tomatoes

1. Place two chicken breasts in each of two large resealable plastic bags. Set them aside.

2. Place the onion, habaneros, lime juice, olive oil, garlic, allspice, thyme, black pepper, nutmeg, and cinnamon in a food processor and pulse until very well blended.

3. Pour half the marinade into each bag with the chicken breasts. Squeeze out as much air as possible, seal the bags, and place them in the refrigerator for 4 hours.

4. Preheat a barbecue to medium-high heat.

5. Let the chicken sit at room temperature for 15 minutes and then grill, turning at least once, until cooked through, about 15 minutes total.

6. Let the chicken rest for about 5 minutes before serving. Divide the greens and tomatoes among four serving plates, and top with the chicken.

COOKING TIP: *If you do not have a barbecue, preheat the oven to 400°F and place the chicken on a baking sheet. Roast the chicken until it's cooked through, turning once, about 15 minutes total.*

Per Serving Calories: 226; Total Fat: 9g; Cholesterol: 81mg; Sodium: 92mg; Total Carbohydrates: 3g; Sugar: 1g; Fiber: 0g; Protein: 33g

Coconut Chicken Curry

CARBS PER SERVING: 15G

SERVES 4 / PREP TIME: 15 MINUTES / COOK TIME: 35 MINUTES

You might think of butter chicken when you sample the creamy rich sauce in this dish, but you'll be happy to know there are fewer calories than in the traditional preparation. Curry can be as hot or mild as you wish; it just depends on the type of curry powder or paste you use in the recipe. You can also serve your curry with sambal oelek or another chili paste so that people eating the curry can adjust the heat to suit their own tastes.

2 teaspoons extra-virgin olive oil

3 (5-ounce) boneless, skinless chicken breasts, cut into 1-inch chunks

1 tablespoon grated fresh ginger

1 tablespoon minced garlic

2 tablespoons curry powder

2 cups low-sodium chicken broth

1 cup canned coconut milk

1 carrot, peeled and diced

1 sweet potato, diced

2 tablespoons chopped fresh cilantro

1. Place a large saucepan over medium-high heat and add the oil.

2. Sauté the chicken until lightly browned and almost cooked through, about 10 minutes.

3. Add the ginger, garlic, and curry powder, and sauté until fragrant, about 3 minutes.

4. Stir in the chicken broth, coconut milk, carrot, and sweet potato and bring the mixture to a boil.

5. Reduce the heat to low and simmer, stirring occasionally, until the vegetables and chicken are tender, about 20 minutes.

6. Stir in the cilantro and serve.

INGREDIENT TIP: *The coconut milk used for the sauce is the thick, creamy product found in cans. Do not use the watery version found in the dairy case or the finished dish won't be as luscious.*

Per Serving Calories: 327; Total Fat: 17g; Cholesterol: 64mg; Sodium: 276mg; Total Carbohydrates: 15g; Sugar: 4g; Fiber: 1g; Protein: 29g

Cheesy Stuffed Chicken Breasts

CARBS PER SERVING: 3G

SERVES 4 / PREP TIME: 15 MINUTES, PLUS 15 MINUTES TO CHILL /
COOK TIME: 30 MINUTES

Black olives add a satisfying saltiness and many health benefits to the chicken filling. Olives are high in monounsaturated fats, antioxidants, iron, vitamin A, and vitamin E and are therefore very good for the heart. Cardiovascular disease risk is often a concern for people with type 2 diabetes, so add some olives to dishes, or enjoy as a snack.

1 cup chopped roasted
red pepper
2 ounces goat cheese
4 Kalamata olives, pitted,
finely chopped
1 tablespoon chopped
fresh basil
4 (5-ounce) boneless, skinless
chicken breasts
1 tablespoon extra-virgin
olive oil

1. Preheat the oven to 400°F.

2. In a small bowl, stir together the red pepper, goat cheese, olives, and basil until well mixed.

3. Place the filling in the refrigerator for about 15 minutes to firm it up.

4. Cut a slit horizontally in each chicken breast to create a pocket in the middle.

5. Evenly divide the filling between the chicken breast pockets and secure them closed with wooden toothpicks.

6. Place a large skillet over medium-high heat and add the olive oil.

7. Brown the chicken breasts on both sides, about 10 minutes in total.

8. Transfer to the oven. Bake the chicken breasts until the chicken is cooked through, about 20 minutes.

9. Let the chicken breasts rest for 10 minutes, remove the toothpicks, and serve.

Per Serving Calories: 245; Total Fat: 9g; Cholesterol: 88mg; Sodium: 279mg;
Total Carbohydrates: 3g; Sugar: 2g; Fiber: 1g; Protein: 35g

Turkey Cabbage Soup

CARBS PER SERVING: 30G

SERVES 4 / PREP TIME: 15 MINUTES / COOK TIME: 30 MINUTES

Soup is pure comfort food, especially when it's bursting with tender chunks of turkey and an assortment of vegetables. Imagine ladling this soup into a large mug and enjoying it while curled up under a fluffy blanket on a chilly fall evening. The turkey can come from a leftover holiday roast, and if you are feeling particularly industrious, you can make the turkey broth from the carcass after the carving is done.

1 tablespoon extra-virgin
    olive oil
1 sweet onion, chopped
2 celery stalks, chopped
2 teaspoons minced
    fresh garlic
4 cups finely shredded
    green cabbage
1 sweet potato, peeled, diced
8 cups chicken or turkey broth
2 bay leaves
1 cup chopped cooked turkey
2 teaspoons chopped
    fresh thyme
Sea salt
Freshly ground black pepper

1. Place a large saucepan over medium-high heat and add the olive oil.

2. Sauté the onion, celery, and garlic until softened and translucent, about 3 minutes.

3. Add the cabbage and sweet potato and sauté for 3 minutes.

4. Stir in the chicken broth and bay leaves and bring the soup to a boil.

5. Reduce the heat to low and simmer until the vegetables are tender, about 20 minutes.

6. Add the turkey and thyme and simmer until the turkey is heated through, about 4 minutes.

7. Remove the bay leaves and season the soup with salt and pepper.

Per Serving Calories: 325; Total Fat: 11g; Cholesterol: 41mg; Sodium: 715mg; Total Carbohydrates: 30g; Sugar: 13g; Fiber: 4g; Protein: 24g

Juicy Turkey Burgers

CARBS PER SERVING: 12G

SERVES 4 / PREP TIME: 10 MINUTES / COOK TIME: 20 MINUTES

Hamburgers are a weekend ritual for some families, so having more than one type in your culinary repertoire is handy. Look for ground turkey that contains both breast and dark meat, if possible, because the flavor is better and the finished burger juicier. These patties freeze well, so double up and store the burgers raw between sheets of parchment in a sealed plastic bag. You can cook them right from frozen.

1½ pounds lean
   ground turkey
½ cup bread crumbs
½ sweet onion, chopped
1 carrot, peeled, grated
1 teaspoon minced garlic
1 teaspoon chopped
   fresh thyme
Sea salt
Freshly ground black pepper
Nonstick cooking spray

1. In a large bowl, mix together the turkey, bread crumbs, onion, carrot, garlic, and thyme until very well mixed.

2. Season the mixture lightly with salt and pepper.

3. Shape the turkey mixture into 4 equal patties.

4. Place a large skillet over medium-high heat and coat it lightly with cooking spray.

5. Cook the turkey patties until golden and completely cooked through, about 10 minutes per side.

6. Serve the burgers plain or with your favorite toppings on a whole-wheat bun.

SUBSTITUTION TIP: *Burgers can be made out of any kind of meat or combination of meats, depending on what is available and your preference. Beef, pork, lamb, chicken, and venison are all wonderful substitutions or additions for this recipe.*

Per Serving Calories: 317; Total Fat: 15g; Cholesterol: 134mg; Sodium: 270mg; Total Carbohydrates: 12g; Sugar: 2g; Fiber: 1g; Protein: 32g

Turkey Stuffed Peppers

CARBS PER SERVING: 14G

SERVES 4 / PREP TIME: 15 MINUTES / COOK TIME: 50 MINUTES

This is a simple, pretty dish, with deep red peppers, flecks of green basil, and snowy feta crumbles. You will be happy to know it is also filled with nutrients to support your health. Red peppers contain a plethora of vitamins and minerals such as vitamin A, vitamin C, niacin, potassium, and folic acid. These rainbow-hued vegetables are also a source of over 30 different carotenoids, which are powerful cancer fighters and provide cardiovascular support.

1 teaspoon extra-virgin olive oil, plus more for greasing the baking dish
1 pound ground turkey breast
½ sweet onion, chopped
1 teaspoon minced garlic
1 tomato, diced
½ teaspoon chopped fresh basil
Sea salt
Freshly ground black pepper
4 red bell peppers, tops cut off, seeded
2 ounces low-sodium feta cheese

1. Preheat the oven to 350°F.

2. Lightly grease a 9-by-9-inch baking dish with olive oil and set it aside.

3. Place a large skillet over medium heat and add 1 teaspoon of olive oil.

4. Add the turkey to the skillet and cook until it is no longer pink, stirring occasionally to break up the meat and brown it evenly, about 6 minutes.

5. Add the onion and garlic and sauté until softened and translucent, about 3 minutes.

6. Stir in the tomato and basil. Season with salt and pepper.

7. Place the peppers cut-side up in the baking dish. Divide the filling into four equal portions and spoon it into the peppers.

8. Sprinkle the feta cheese on top of the filling.

9. Add ¼ cup of water to the dish and cover with aluminum foil.

10. Bake the peppers until they are soft and heated through, about 40 minutes.

Per Serving Calories: 280; Total Fat: 14g; Cholesterol: 102mg; Sodium: 271mg; Total Carbohydrates: 14g; Sugar: 9g; Fiber: 4g; Protein: 24g

Herb-Roasted Turkey and Vegetables

CARBS PER SERVING: 20G

SERVES 6 / PREP TIME: 20 MINUTES / COOK TIME: 2 HOURS

Turkey is not just for holidays and can certainly be part of a regular weekday meal, especially if it means there are leftovers for lunch the next day. Turkey is high in potassium, protein, selenium, zinc, and iron, as well as B vitamins. This combination of nutrients can cut the risk of some cancers and fight free radicals, helping reduce poor blood flow and limit the complications associated with diabetes.

2 teaspoons minced garlic

1 tablespoon chopped fresh parsley

1 teaspoon chopped fresh thyme

1 teaspoon chopped fresh rosemary

2 pounds boneless, skinless whole turkey breast

3 teaspoons extra-virgin olive oil, divided

Sea salt

Freshly ground black pepper

2 sweet potatoes, peeled and cut into 2-inch chunks

2 carrots, peeled and cut into 2-inch chunks

2 parsnips, peeled and cut into 2-inch chunks

1 sweet onion, peeled and cut into eighths

1. Preheat the oven to 350°F.

2. Line a large roasting pan with aluminum foil and set it aside.

3. In a small bowl, mix together the garlic, parsley, thyme, and rosemary.

4. Place the turkey breast in the roasting pan and rub it all over with 1 teaspoon of olive oil.

5. Rub the garlic-herb mixture all over the turkey and season lightly with salt and pepper.

6. Place the turkey in the oven and roast for 30 minutes.

7. While the turkey is roasting, toss the sweet potatoes, carrots, parsnips, onion, and the remaining 2 teaspoons of olive oil in a large bowl.

8. Remove the turkey from the oven and arrange the vegetables around it.

9. Roast until the turkey is cooked through (170°F internal temperature) and the vegetables are lightly caramelized, about 1½ hours.

COOKING TIP: *If you want lots of leftovers, double this recipe and use the extra meat for a fabulous soup, or pile it on whole-grain bread for a healthy sandwich.*

Per Serving Calories: 273; Total Fat: 3g; Cholesterol: 93mg; Sodium: 116mg; Total Carbohydrates: 20g; Sugar: 6g; Fiber: 4g; Protein: 38g

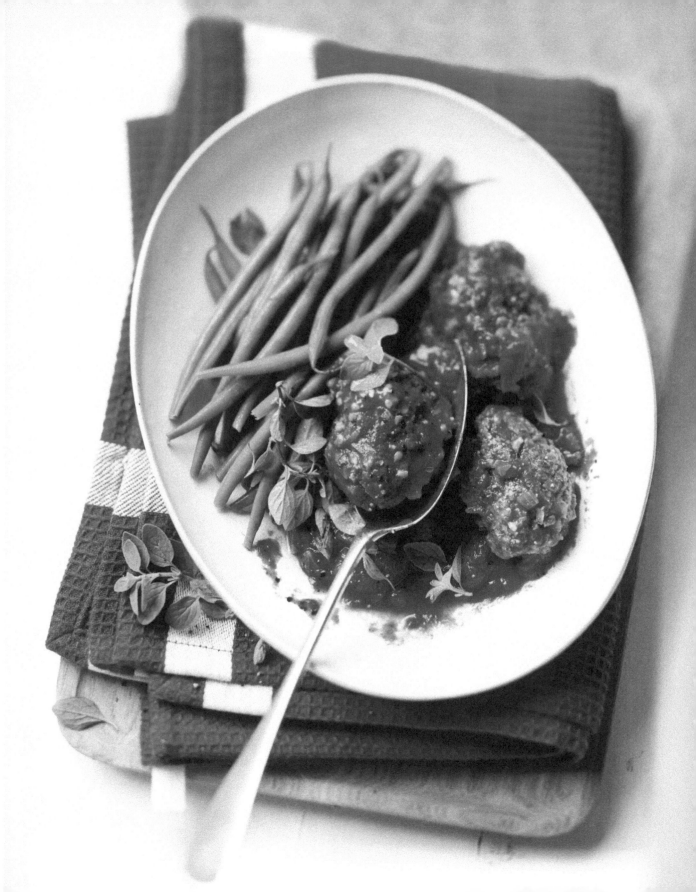

CHAPTER 6

Pork, Lamb, and Beef Mains

Pork Chop Diane

CARBS PER SERVING: 1G

SERVES 4 / PREP TIME: 10 MINUTES / COOK TIME: 20 MINUTES

Pork is often overlooked when people are thinking about meat for a nutritious main meal. Pork is very lean and has fewer calories than poultry or beef, especially if you trim any visible fat from the chops and choose a healthy cooking method such as roasting or grilling. Thick pork tenderloin slices would also be a nice choice for this recipe, if you are not in the mood for pork chops.

¼ cup low-sodium chicken broth

1 tablespoon freshly squeezed lemon juice

2 teaspoons Worcestershire sauce

2 teaspoons Dijon mustard

4 (5-ounce) boneless pork top loin chops, about 1 inch thick

Sea salt

Freshly ground black pepper

1 teaspoon extra-virgin olive oil

1 teaspoon lemon zest

1 teaspoon butter

2 teaspoons chopped fresh chives

1. In a small bowl, stir together the chicken broth, lemon juice, Worcestershire sauce, and Dijon mustard and set it aside.

2. Season the pork chops lightly with salt and pepper.

3. Place a large skillet over medium-high heat and add the olive oil.

4. Cook the pork chops, turning once, until they are no longer pink, about 8 minutes per side.

5. Transfer the chops to a plate and set it aside.

6. Pour the broth mixture into the skillet and cook until warmed through and thickened, about 2 minutes.

7. Whisk in the lemon zest, butter, and chives.

8. Serve the chops with a generous spoonful of sauce.

Per Serving Calories: 200; Total Fat: 8g; Cholesterol: 70mg; Sodium: 394mg; Total Carbohydrates: 1g; Sugar: 1g; Fiber: 0g; Protein: 30g

Autumn Pork Chops with Red Cabbage and Apples

CARBS PER SERVING: 12G

SERVES 4 / PREP TIME: 15 MINUTES / COOK TIME: 30 MINUTES

Your grandmother might have served a meal very similar to this if she lived on a farm and grew apples and cabbage. Humble, simple, and tasty: good food certainly does not need to be time-consuming or contain complicated ingredients. Take the time to brown the pork chops to a pretty golden color all over, because you will be cooking the rest of the ingredients in the same skillet and little caramelized bits of pork add to the overall taste of the meal.

¼ cup apple cider vinegar

2 tablespoons granulated sweetener

4 (4-ounce) pork chops, about 1 inch thick

Sea salt

Freshly ground black pepper

1 tablespoon extra-virgin olive oil

½ red cabbage, finely shredded

1 sweet onion, thinly sliced

1 apple, peeled, cored, and sliced

1 teaspoon chopped fresh thyme

1. In a small bowl, whisk together the vinegar and sweetener. Set it aside.

2. Season the pork with salt and pepper.

3. Place a large skillet over medium-high heat and add the olive oil.

4. Cook the pork chops until no longer pink, turning once, about 8 minutes per side.

5. Transfer the chops to a plate and set aside.

6. Add the cabbage and onion to the skillet and sauté until the vegetables have softened, about 5 minutes.

7. Add the vinegar mixture and the apple slices to the skillet and bring the mixture to a boil.

8. Reduce the heat to low and simmer, covered, for 5 additional minutes.

9. Return the pork chops to the skillet, along with any accumulated juices and thyme, cover, and cook for 5 more minutes.

Per Serving Calories: 223; Total Fat: 8g; Cholesterol: 54mg; Sodium: 292mg; Total Carbohydrates: 12g; Sugar: 8g; Fiber: 3g; Protein: 26g

Chipotle Chili Pork Chops

CARBS PER SERVING: 1G

SERVES 4 / PREP TIME: 5 MINUTES, PLUS 4 HOURS TO MARINATE / COOK TIME: 20 MINUTES

The best way to cook your fiery chipotle chops is on the barbecue, although the oven works well too. If you're barbecuing, consider throwing thick slices of oil-tossed sweet potato on the grill as an accompaniment, or stalks of tender asparagus. These spicy chops would be fantastic sliced up in a wrap for lunch the next day.

Juice and zest of 1 lime
1 tablespoon extra-virgin olive oil
1 tablespoon chipotle chili powder
2 teaspoons minced garlic
1 teaspoon ground cinnamon
Pinch sea salt
4 (5-ounce) pork chops, about 1 inch thick
Lime wedges, for garnish

1. Combine the lime juice and zest, oil, chipotle chili powder, garlic, cinnamon, and salt in a resealable plastic bag. Add the pork chops. Remove as much air as possible and seal the bag.

2. Marinate the chops in the refrigerator for at least 4 hours, and up to 24 hours, turning them several times.

3. Preheat the oven to 400°F and set a rack on a baking sheet. Let the chops rest at room temperature for 15 minutes, then arrange them on the rack and discard the remaining marinade.

4. Roast the chops until cooked through, turning once, about 10 minutes per side.

5. Serve with lime wedges.

INGREDIENT TIP: *Chipotle chili powder is not the same as regular chili powder, so try to find it for this dish, as it has a richer, more complex, intoxicating smoky taste.*

Per Serving Calories: 204; Total Fat: 9g; Cholesterol: 67mg; Sodium: 317mg; Total Carbohydrates: 1g; Sugar: 1g; Fiber: 0g; Protein: 30g

Orange-Marinated Pork Tenderloin

CARBS PER SERVING: 4G

SERVES 4 / PREP TIME: 10 MINUTES, PLUS 2 HOURS TO MARINATE /
COOK TIME: 30 MINUTES

Pork tenderloin is like a small roast that can be sliced into perfect juicy rounds. Trimmed pork tenderloin is incredibly lean, because all the fat and the silver skin are carefully sliced off, leaving only meat. Silver skin is a tough connective tissue that does not dissolve when the meat is cooked. Try to buy this cut already cleaned, because you need a very sharp knife and a steady hand to remove the silver skin effectively.

¼ cup freshly squeezed orange juice
2 teaspoons orange zest
2 teaspoons minced garlic
1 teaspoon low-sodium soy sauce
1 teaspoon grated fresh ginger
1 teaspoon honey
1½ pounds pork tenderloin roast, trimmed of fat
1 tablespoon extra-virgin olive oil

1. In a small bowl, whisk together the orange juice, zest, garlic, soy sauce, ginger, and honey.

2. Pour the marinade into a resealable plastic bag and add the pork tenderloin.

3. Remove as much air as possible and seal the bag. Marinate the pork in the refrigerator, turning the bag a few times, for 2 hours.

4. Preheat the oven to 400°F.

5. Remove the tenderloin from the marinade and discard the marinade.

6. Place a large ovenproof skillet over medium-high heat and add the oil.

7. Sear the pork tenderloin on all sides, about 5 minutes in total.

8. Transfer the skillet to the oven and roast the pork until just cooked through, about 25 minutes.

9. Let the meat stand for 10 minutes before serving.

COOKING TIP: *Leftover pork is a perfect wrap or pita filling. To create a spectacular lunch treat with a subtle Asian flavor, add shredded cucumber, crispy red bell pepper strips, and a dash of hot sauce to the pork.*

Per Serving Calories: 228; Total Fat: 9g; Cholesterol: 82mg; Sodium: 486mg; Total Carbohydrates: 4g; Sugar: 3g; Fiber: 0g; Protein: 34g

Homestyle Herb Meatballs

CARBS PER SERVING: 13G

SERVES 4 / PREP TIME: 10 MINUTES / COOK TIME: 15 MINUTES

Making good meatballs is close to an art and a tremendous source of pride for many home cooks. Meatballs need a cohesive blend of meat, herbs, and, in some cases, fat to create a tender finished product rather than tough, tasteless chunks of ground meat. This recipe is light on fat but uses an egg to bring it all together for meatballs you'll be proud of.

½ pound lean ground pork
½ pound lean ground beef
1 sweet onion, finely chopped
¼ cup bread crumbs
2 tablespoons chopped
    fresh basil
2 teaspoons minced garlic
1 egg
Pinch sea salt
Pinch freshly ground
    black pepper

1. Preheat the oven to 350°F.

2. Line a baking tray with parchment paper and set it aside.

3. In a large bowl, mix together the pork, beef, onion, bread crumbs, basil, garlic, egg, salt, and pepper until very well mixed.

4. Roll the meat mixture into 2-inch meatballs.

5. Transfer the meatballs to the baking sheet and bake until they are browned and cooked through, about 15 minutes.

6. Serve the meatballs with your favorite marinara sauce and some steamed green beans.

COOKING TIP: *If you are going to save some time in the kitchen by making your meals ahead, this recipe is a perfect choice. You can freeze the meatballs either raw or cooked, depending on which dishes you want to make during the week.*

Per Serving Calories: 332; Total Fat: 19g; Cholesterol: 130mg; Sodium: 188mg; Total Carbohydrates: 13g; Sugar: 3g; Fiber: 1g; Protein: 24g

Lime-Parsley Lamb Cutlets

CARBS PER SERVING: 1G

SERVES 4 / PREP TIME: 10 MINUTES, PLUS 4 HOURS TO MARINATE /
COOK TIME: 10 MINUTES

Parsley is not just a garnish that you toss to the edge of your plate. It is a nutrient-packed herb that has been used in many cuisines for centuries. Parsley is a wonderful source of flavonoids such as luteolin, vitamin K, vitamin C, folate, and iron. Eating parsley regularly can protect your body against stroke, heart disease, cancer, and rheumatoid arthritis. Either curly or Italian flat-leaf parsley will work with these citrusy chops.

¼ cup extra-virgin olive oil
¼ cup freshly squeezed
    lime juice
2 tablespoons lime zest
2 tablespoons chopped
    fresh parsley
Pinch sea salt
Pinch freshly ground
    black pepper
12 lamb cutlets (about
    1½ pounds total)

1. In a medium bowl, whisk together the oil, lime juice, zest, parsley, salt, and pepper.

2. Transfer the marinade to a resealable plastic bag.

3. Add the cutlets to the bag and remove as much air as possible before sealing.

4. Marinate the lamb in the refrigerator for about 4 hours, turning the bag several times.

5. Preheat the oven to broil.

6. Remove the chops from the bag and arrange them on an aluminum foil–lined baking sheet. Discard the marinade.

7. Broil the chops for 4 minutes per side for medium doneness.

8. Let the chops rest for 5 minutes before serving.

Per Serving Calories: 413; Total Fat: 29g; Cholesterol: 111mg; Sodium: 100mg; Total Carbohydrates: 1g; Sugar: 0g; Fiber: 0g; Protein: 31g

Spiced Lamb Stew

CARBS PER SERVING: 16G

SERVES 4 / PREP TIME: 20 MINUTES / COOK TIME: 2 HOURS, 15 MINUTES

Tender chunks of lamb accented with sweet potato and warm spices seems like a North African–influenced meal. But lamb is very popular in many other countries, especially where there are limited or unsuitable grazing lands. Look for local lamb and, whenever possible, organic meat, because it has more nutrients than commercially raised lamb. Natural organic lamb has a high omega-3 content and is leaner as well.

2 tablespoons extra-virgin olive oil

1½ pounds lamb shoulder, cut into 1-inch chunks

½ sweet onion, chopped

1 tablespoon grated fresh ginger

2 teaspoons minced garlic

1 teaspoon ground cinnamon

1 teaspoon ground cumin

¼ teaspoon ground cloves

2 sweet potatoes, peeled, diced

2 cups low-sodium beef broth

Sea salt

Freshly ground back pepper

2 teaspoons chopped fresh parsley, for garnish

1. Preheat the oven to 300°F.

2. Place a large ovenproof skillet over medium-high heat and add the olive oil.

3. Brown the lamb, stirring occasionally, for about 6 minutes.

4. Add the onion, ginger, garlic, cinnamon, cumin, and cloves, and sauté for 5 minutes.

5. Add the sweet potatoes and beef broth and bring the stew to a boil.

6. Cover the skillet and transfer the lamb to the oven. Braise, stirring occasionally, until the lamb is very tender, about 2 hours.

7. Remove the stew from the oven and season with salt and pepper.

8. Serve garnished with the parsley.

SUBSTITUTION TIP: *Sometimes lamb is unavailable or not the right cut for a delicious hearty stew. If you can't find this tender meat, try using the same amount of beef or pork instead.*

Per Serving Calories: 545; Total Fat: 35g; Cholesterol: 109mg; Sodium: 395mg; Total Carbohydrates: 16g; Sugar: 4g; Fiber: 2g; Protein: 32g

Beef Barley Soup

CARBS PER SERVING: 33G

SERVES 4 / PREP TIME: 20 MINUTES / COOK TIME: 30 MINUTES

Barley is a cereal grain with a unique nutty taste and slightly chewy texture that is marvelous in soups and stews, but is often underused. It is an excellent source of manganese, copper, fiber, selenium, and chromium. It's high in fiber and can keep your digestive system in tip-top shape while lowering cholesterol and cutting the risk of colon cancer. The insoluble fiber in this grain is a food source for the friendly bacteria found in the gut that can crowd out pathological bacteria. Try to include barley at least once a week in your meal plans.

2 teaspoons extra-virgin olive oil
1 sweet onion, chopped
1 tablespoon minced garlic
4 celery stalks, with greens, chopped
2 carrots, peeled, diced
1 sweet potato, peeled, diced
8 cups low-sodium beef broth
1 cup cooked pearl barley
2 cups diced cooked beef
2 bay leaves
2 teaspoons hot sauce
2 teaspoons chopped fresh thyme
1 cup shredded kale
Sea salt
Freshly ground black pepper

1. Place a large stockpot over medium-high heat and add the oil.

2. Sauté the onion and garlic until softened and translucent, about 3 minutes.

3. Stir in the celery, carrot, and sweet potato, and sauté for a further 5 minutes.

4. Stir in the beef broth, barley, beef, bay leaves, and hot sauce.

5. Bring the soup to a boil, then reduce the heat to low.

6. Simmer until the vegetables are tender, about 15 minutes.

7. Remove the bay leaves and stir in the thyme and kale.

8. Simmer for 5 minutes, and season with salt and pepper.

COOKING TIP: *This soup is so quick to prepare because the beef and barley are already cooked when they go in with the rest of the ingredients. Cook these items ahead and freeze them in the right amounts in resealable freezer bags.*

Per Serving Calories: 345; Total Fat: 11g; Cholesterol: 30mg; Sodium: 837mg; Total Carbohydrates: 33g; Sugar: 8g; Fiber: 5g; Protein: 28g

Mediterranean Steak Sandwiches

CARBS PER SERVING: 22G

SERVES 4 / PREP TIME: 10 MINUTES, PLUS 1 HOUR TO MARINATE /
COOK TIME: 10 MINUTES

The marinated steak used in this pita sandwich is a perfect choice for dinner: The fresh salad is included. Or skip the pita and serve the steak with a delightful rice or grain side dish and some vegetables. Try cooking two steaks and keeping one for lunch the next day, when a Mediterranean-flavored sandwich will provide tons of energy and keep you going until dinner.

2 tablespoons extra-virgin
    olive oil
2 tablespoons
    balsamic vinegar
2 teaspoons minced garlic
2 teaspoons freshly squeezed
    lemon juice
2 teaspoons chopped
    fresh oregano
1 teaspoon chopped
    fresh parsley
1 pound flank steak, trimmed
    of fat
4 whole-wheat pitas
2 cups shredded lettuce
1 red onion, thinly sliced
1 tomato, chopped
1 ounce low-sodium
    feta cheese

1. In a large bowl, whisk together the olive oil, balsamic vinegar, garlic, lemon juice, oregano, and parsley.

2. Add the steak to the bowl, turning to coat it completely.

3. Marinate the steak for 1 hour in the refrigerator, turning it over several times.

4. Preheat the broiler. Line a baking sheet with aluminum foil.

5. Take the steak out of the bowl and discard the marinade.

6. Place the steak on the baking sheet and broil until it is done to your liking, about 5 minutes per side for medium.

7. Let the steak rest for 10 minutes before slicing it thinly on a bias.

8. Stuff the pitas with the sliced steak, lettuce, onion, tomato, and feta.

Per Serving Calories: 344; Total Fat: 16g; Cholesterol: 53mg; Sodium: 296mg; Total Carbohydrates: 22g; Sugar: 3g; Fiber: 3g; Protein: 28g

Roasted Beef with Peppercorn Sauce

CARBS PER SERVING: 4G

SERVES 4 / PREP TIME: 10 MINUTES / COOK TIME: 1 HOUR, 40 MINUTES

Peppercorn sauce is an extremely popular choice for steak in high-end restaurants because the heat from the pepper wakes up the palate and highlights the taste of the beef. Green peppercorns are found in tiny cans in the condiment section of your grocery store; you will probably not use the entire amount for this recipe unless you double up on the sauce. Transfer the remaining peppercorns and the brine in the can to a small sealable plastic container for storing.

1½ pounds top rump
    beef roast
Sea salt
Freshly ground black pepper
3 teaspoons extra-virgin olive
    oil, divided
3 shallots, minced
2 teaspoons minced garlic
1 tablespoon
    green peppercorns
2 tablespoons dry sherry
2 tablespoons all-
    purpose flour
1 cup sodium-free beef broth

1. Heat the oven to 300°F.

2. Season the roast with salt and pepper.

3. Place a large skillet over medium-high heat and add 2 teaspoons of olive oil.

4. Brown the beef on all sides, about 10 minutes in total, and transfer the roast to a baking dish.

5. Roast until desired doneness, about 1½ hours for medium. When the roast has been in the oven for 1 hour, start the sauce.

6. In a medium saucepan over medium-high heat, sauté the shallots in the remaining 1 teaspoon of olive oil until translucent, about 4 minutes.

7. Stir in the garlic and peppercorns, and cook for another minute. Whisk in the sherry to deglaze the pan.

8. Whisk in the flour to form a thick paste, cooking for 1 minute and stirring constantly.

9. Pour in the beef broth and whisk until the sauce is thick and glossy, about 4 minutes. Season the sauce with salt and pepper.

10. Serve the beef with a generous spoonful of sauce.

Per Serving Calories: 330; Total Fat: 18g; Cholesterol: 109mg; Sodium: 207mg; Total Carbohydrates: 4g; Sugar: 1g; Fiber: 0g; Protein: 36g

Coffee-and-Herb-Marinated Steak

CARBS PER SERVING: 0G

SERVES 4 / PREP TIME: 10 MINUTES, PLUS 2 HOURS TO MARINATE /
COOK TIME: 10 MINUTES

Coffee might seem like a strange ingredient to find in a meat marinade, but it is perfect if you enjoy a slightly smoky flavor and do not want to use chemicals such as liquid smoke to get it. Your dinner guests will never guess what that indefinable savory flavor taste is in their steak. You can also use cold coffee, so save your leftover brewed coffee from breakfast. Just substitute about 1 cup for the coffee beans, and add it with the oil and vinegar in step 2.

¼ cup whole coffee beans

2 teaspoons minced garlic

2 teaspoons chopped
  fresh rosemary

2 teaspoons chopped
  fresh thyme

1 teaspoon freshly ground
  black pepper

2 tablespoons apple
  cider vinegar

2 tablespoons extra-virgin
  olive oil

1 pound flank steak, trimmed
  of visible fat

1. Place the coffee beans, garlic, rosemary, thyme, and black pepper in a coffee grinder or food processor and pulse until coarsely ground.

2. Transfer the coffee mixture to a resealable plastic bag and add the vinegar and oil. Shake to combine.

3. Add the flank steak and squeeze the excess air out of the bag. Seal it. Marinate the steak in the refrigerator for at least 2 hours, occasionally turning the bag over.

4. Preheat the broiler. Line a baking sheet with aluminum foil.

5. Take the steak out of the bowl and discard the marinade.

6. Place the steak on the baking sheet and broil until it is done to your liking, about 5 minutes per side for medium.

7. Let the steak rest for 10 minutes before slicing it thinly on a bias.

8. Serve with a mixed green salad or your favorite side dish.

INGREDIENT TIP: *There is nothing like the fragrance of fresh ground coffee, even if you aren't a coffee drinker. Get dark robust coffee beans for this marinade to bring out the flavor of the steak.*

Per Serving Calories: 313; Total Fat: 20g; Cholesterol: 61mg; Sodium: 79mg; Total Carbohydrates: 0g; Sugar: 0g; Fiber: 0g; Protein: 31g

Traditional Beef Stroganoff

CARBS PER SERVING: 6G

SERVES 4 / PREP TIME: 10 MINUTES / COOK TIME: 30 MINUTES

Caramelized mushrooms provide much of the tantalizing flavor of this classic preparation. Mushrooms are a good source of vitamin D, which fruits and vegetables do not contain. Vitamin D is particularly important for people with type 2 diabetes because a deficiency is linked to an increased risk of glucose intolerance. Mushrooms are also high in B vitamins, iron, and many antioxidants, so enjoy this dish regularly for all its taste and health benefits.

1 teaspoon extra-virgin olive oil

1 pound top sirloin, cut into thin strips

1 cup sliced button mushrooms

½ sweet onion, finely chopped

1 teaspoon minced garlic

1 tablespoon whole-wheat flour

½ cup low-sodium beef broth

¼ cup dry sherry

½ cup fat-free sour cream

1 tablespoon chopped fresh parsley

Sea salt

Freshly ground black pepper

1. Place a large skillet over medium-high heat and add the oil.

2. Sauté the beef until browned, about 10 minutes, then remove the beef with a slotted spoon to a plate and set it aside.

3. Add the mushrooms, onion, and garlic to the skillet and sauté until lightly browned, about 5 minutes.

4. Whisk in the flour and then whisk in the beef broth and sherry.

5. Return the sirloin to the skillet and bring the mixture to a boil.

6. Reduce the heat to low and simmer until the beef is tender, about 10 minutes.

7. Stir in the sour cream and parsley. Season with salt and pepper.

Per Serving Calories: 257; Total Fat: 14g; Cholesterol: 48mg; Sodium: 141mg; Total Carbohydrates: 6g; Sugar: 1g; Fiber: 1g; Protein: 26g

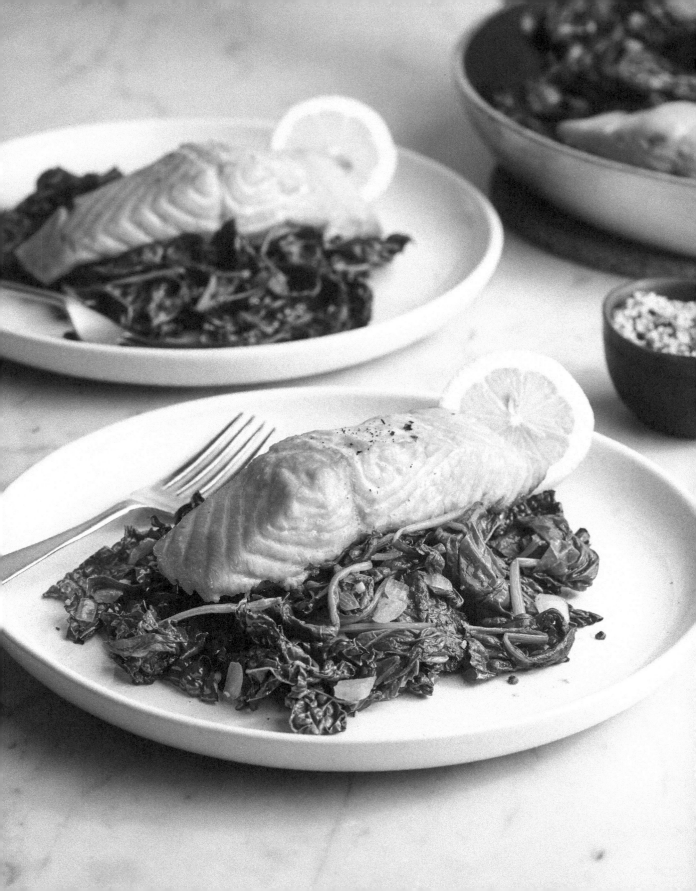

CHAPTER 7

Fish and Seafood Mains

Shrimp with Tomatoes and Feta

CARBS PER SERVING: 12G

SERVES 4 / PREP TIME: 10 MINUTES / COOK TIME: 30 MINUTES

Shrimp and tomatoes are an inspired combination because they are both sweet and cook quickly. You can buy your shrimp cleaned to save time, or do it yourself to save money. Frozen shrimp might be a good option because most are flash-frozen within an hour of being caught. Goat cheese would be a delightful substitute for feta here; look for a semisoft product so that it crumbles easily.

3 tomatoes, coarsely chopped
½ cup chopped
    sun-dried tomatoes
2 teaspoons minced garlic
2 teaspoons extra-virgin
    olive oil
1 teaspoon chopped
    fresh oregano
Freshly ground black pepper
1½ pounds (16–20 count)
    shrimp, peeled, deveined,
    tails removed
4 teaspoons freshly squeezed
    lemon juice
½ cup low-sodium feta
    cheese, crumbled

1. Heat the oven to 450°F.

2. In a medium bowl, toss the tomatoes, sun-dried tomatoes, garlic, oil, and oregano until well combined.

3. Season the mixture lightly with pepper.

4. Transfer the tomato mixture to a 9-by-13-inch glass baking dish.

5. Bake until softened, about 15 minutes.

6. Stir the shrimp and lemon juice into the hot tomato mixture and top evenly with the feta.

7. Bake until the shrimp are cooked through, about 15 minutes more.

INGREDIENT TIP: *Shrimp are sold by size, using the measurement unit of count per pound. So 16–20 count means there are 16 to 20 shrimp in a pound. The higher the number, the smaller the shrimp. If you want this meal ready quicker, switch to smaller 36–40 count shrimp, and cut the cooking time for the shrimp to about 7 minutes.*

Per Serving Calories: 306; Total Fat: 11g; Cholesterol: 272mg; Sodium: 502mg; Total Carbohydrates: 12g; Sugar: 5g; Fiber: 3g; Protein: 39g

Orange-Infused Scallops

CARBS PER SERVING: 8G

SERVES 4 / PREP TIME: 10 MINUTES / COOK TIME: 10 MINUTES

Scallops are a convenient choice for anyone who wants a quick, healthy meal because they are available frozen year-round and cook in less than 10 minutes. Scallops are low-calorie, low-fat, and high in protein, iodine, omega-3 fatty acids, magnesium, and vitamin B_{12}. These sweet, tender mollusks can reduce the risk of cardiovascular disease, cancer, and stroke. Make sure you cook your scallops within one day after buying or thawing them, because they perish quickly.

2 pounds sea scallops
Sea salt
Freshly ground black pepper
2 tablespoons extra-virgin olive oil
1 tablespoon minced garlic
¼ cup freshly squeezed orange juice
1 teaspoon orange zest
2 teaspoons chopped fresh thyme, for garnish

1. Clean the scallops and pat them dry with paper towels, then season them lightly with salt and pepper.

2. Place a large skillet over medium-high heat and add the olive oil.

3. Sauté the garlic until it is softened and translucent, about 3 minutes.

4. Add the scallops to the skillet and cook until they are lightly seared and just cooked through, turning once, about 4 minutes per side.

5. Transfer the scallops to a plate, cover to keep warm, and set them aside.

6. Add the orange juice and zest to the skillet and stir to scrape up any cooked bits.

7. Spoon the sauce over the scallops and serve, garnished with the thyme.

Per Serving Calories: 267; Total Fat: 8g; Cholesterol: 74mg; Sodium: 361mg; Total Carbohydrates: 8g; Sugar: 1g; Fiber: 0g; Protein: 38g

Crab Cakes with Honeydew Melon Salsa

CARBS PER SERVING: 18G

SERVES 4 / PREP TIME: 30 MINUTES, PLUS 1 HOUR TO CHILL / COOK TIME: 10 MINUTES

Crab cakes are an ideal meal for summer, or when you want to be reminded of balmy days. These light, sweet, golden nuggets are low in fat and calories while being high in protein and vitamin B_{12}. Including crab as a regular part of your diet supports brain function and protects against heart disease, but since this shellfish is also higher in sodium and cholesterol than some other seafoods, don't go overboard!

FOR THE SALSA
1 cup finely chopped
    honeydew melon
1 scallion, white and green
    parts, finely chopped
1 red bell pepper, seeded,
    finely chopped
1 teaspoon chopped
    fresh thyme
Pinch sea salt
Pinch freshly ground
    black pepper

FOR THE CRAB CAKES
1 pound lump crabmeat,
    drained and picked over
¼ cup finely chopped
    red onion
¼ cup panko bread crumbs
1 tablespoon chopped
    fresh parsley
1 teaspoon lemon zest
1 egg
¼ cup whole-wheat flour
Nonstick cooking spray

TO MAKE THE SALSA

1. In a small bowl, stir together the melon, scallion, bell pepper, and thyme.

2. Season the salsa with salt and pepper and set aside.

TO MAKE THE CRAB CAKES

1. In a medium bowl, mix together the crab, onion, bread crumbs, parsley, lemon zest, and egg until very well combined.

2. Divide the crab mixture into 8 equal portions and form them into patties about ¾-inch thick.

3. Chill the crab cakes in the refrigerator for at least 1 hour to firm them up.

4. Dredge the chilled crab cakes in the flour until lightly coated, shaking off any excess flour.

5. Place a large skillet over medium heat and lightly coat it with cooking spray.

6. Cook the crab cakes until they are golden brown, turning once, about 5 minutes per side.

7. Serve warm with the salsa.

COOKING TIP: *Crab cakes freeze beautifully, so make a double batch to enjoy later. Freeze them between sheets of parchment paper in a resealable container, for up to 1 month.*

Per Serving Calories: 232; Total Fat: 3g; Cholesterol: 137mg; Sodium: 767mg; Total Carbohydrates: 18g; Sugar: 6g; Fiber: 2g; Protein: 32g

Seafood Stew

CARBS PER SERVING: 19G

SERVES 6 / PREP TIME: 20 MINUTES / COOK TIME: 30 MINUTES

Stew has many different components, from the main proteins to herbs and vegetables. Each ingredient adds something to the final dish, and humble celery is no exception. Celery is a wonderful source of potassium, calcium, coumarins, magnesium, and vitamin C. This crisp vegetable can help lower blood pressure, which can be an issue for people with type 2 diabetes. Celery is a cancer fighter and boosts the immune system. Make sure you include the leafy tops for extra flavor and nutritional impact.

1 tablespoon extra-virgin olive oil
1 sweet onion, chopped
2 teaspoons minced garlic
3 celery stalks, chopped
2 carrots, peeled and chopped
1 (28-ounce) can sodium-free diced tomatoes, undrained
3 cups low-sodium chicken broth
½ cup clam juice
¼ cup dry white wine
2 teaspoons chopped fresh basil
2 teaspoons chopped fresh oregano
2 (4-ounce) haddock fillets, cut into 1-inch chunks
1 pound mussels, scrubbed, debearded
8 ounces (16–20 count) shrimp, peeled, deveined, quartered
Sea salt
Freshly ground black pepper
2 tablespoons chopped fresh parsley

1. Place a large saucepan over medium-high heat and add the olive oil.

2. Sauté the onion and garlic until softened and translucent, about 3 minutes.

3. Stir in the celery and carrots and sauté for 4 minutes.

4. Stir in the tomatoes, chicken broth, clam juice, white wine, basil, and oregano.

5. Bring the sauce to a boil, then reduce the heat to low. Simmer for 15 minutes.

6. Add the fish and mussels, cover, and cook until the mussels open, about 5 minutes.

7. Discard any unopened mussels. Add the shrimp to the pan and cook until the shrimp are opaque, about 2 minutes.

8. Season with salt and pepper. Serve garnished with the chopped parsley.

Per Serving Calories: 248; Total Fat: 7g; Cholesterol: 103mg; Sodium: 577mg; Total Carbohydrates: 19g; Sugar: 7g; Fiber: 2g; Protein: 28g

Sole Piccata

CARBS PER SERVING: 7G

SERVES 4 / PREP TIME: 10 MINUTES / COOK TIME: 20 MINUTES

You will feel like a four-star chef when whipping up this speedy, professional-tasting dish. Choose a quick side dish, such as roasted asparagus or a simple mixed vegetable sauté, so your meal is not delayed by preparing the sides. When purchasing the sole, ask to smell the fillets to ensure their freshness. The fish should have no discernible fishy aroma and the texture should be firm, with no mushy-looking areas.

1 teaspoon extra-virgin olive oil

4 (5-ounce) sole fillets, patted dry

3 tablespoons butter

2 teaspoons minced garlic

2 tablespoons all-purpose flour

2 cups low-sodium chicken broth

Juice and zest of ½ lemon

2 tablespoons capers

1. Place a large skillet over medium-high heat and add the olive oil.

2. Pat the sole fillets dry with paper towels then pan-sear them until the fish flakes easily when tested with a fork, about 4 minutes on each side. Transfer the fish to a plate and set it aside.

3. Return the skillet to the stove and add the butter.

4. Sauté the garlic until translucent, about 3 minutes.

5. Whisk in the flour to make a thick paste and cook, stirring constantly, until the mixture is golden brown, about 2 minutes.

6. Whisk in the chicken broth, lemon juice, and lemon zest.

7. Cook until the sauce has thickened, about 4 minutes.

8. Stir in the capers and serve the sauce over the fish.

INGREDIENT TIP: *Capers are unripened flower buds that are usually brined or dried. They have a citrusy, olive-like flavor. They can usually be found in jars in the pickle or condiment section of the supermarket.*

Per Serving Calories: 271; Total Fat: 13g; Cholesterol: 94mg; Sodium: 413mg; Total Carbohydrates: 7g; Sugar: 2g; Fiber: 0g; Protein: 30g

Spicy Citrus Sole

CARBS PER SERVING: 0G

SERVES 4 / PREP TIME: 10 MINUTES / COOK TIME: 10 MINUTES

Spice rubs are a convenient and delicious way to impart flavor to whatever protein you are cooking, including this popular fish. If you enjoy the combination of spices and zest in this recipe, double or triple the spice rub and keep the mixture in the refrigerator in a sealed container for up to two weeks. The lemon zest and lime zest will dry out, but they'll still pack a strong citrus punch.

1 teaspoon chili powder
1 teaspoon garlic powder
½ teaspoon lime zest
½ teaspoon lemon zest
¼ teaspoon freshly ground black pepper
¼ teaspoon smoked paprika
Pinch sea salt
4 (6-ounce) sole fillets, patted dry
1 tablespoon extra-virgin olive oil
2 teaspoons freshly squeezed lime juice

1. Preheat the oven to 450°F.

2. Line a baking sheet with aluminum foil and set it aside.

3. In a small bowl, stir together the chili powder, garlic powder, lime zest, lemon zest, pepper, paprika, and salt until well mixed.

4. Pat the fish fillets dry with paper towels, place them on the baking sheet, and rub them lightly all over with the spice mixture.

5. Drizzle the olive oil and lime juice on the top of the fish.

6. Bake until the fish flakes when pressed lightly with a fork, about 8 minutes. Serve immediately.

Per Serving Calories: 184; Total Fat: 5g; Cholesterol: 81mg; Sodium: 137mg; Total Carbohydrates: 0g; Sugar: 0g; Fiber: 0g; Protein: 32g

Haddock with Creamy Cucumber Sauce

CARBS PER SERVING: 4G

SERVES 4 / PREP TIME: 10 MINUTES / COOK TIME: 10 MINUTES

Haddock is often served encased in crispy beer batter and surrounded by French fries—which is delicious but very unhealthy. This snowy, mild fish flakes off in delectable juicy chunks when cooked and is an extremely nutritious choice when it isn't deep-fried. The creamy sauce can be made ahead and kept in the fridge in a sealed container for up to three days.

¼ cup 2 percent plain Greek yogurt

½ English cucumber, grated, liquid squeezed out

½ scallion, white and green parts, finely chopped

2 teaspoons chopped fresh mint

1 teaspoon honey

Sea salt

4 (5-ounce) haddock fillets

Freshly ground black pepper

Nonstick cooking spray

1. In a small bowl, stir together the yogurt, cucumber, scallion, mint, honey, and a pinch of salt. Set it aside.

2. Pat the fish fillets dry with paper towels and season them lightly with salt and pepper.

3. Place a large skillet over medium-high heat and spray lightly with cooking spray.

4. Cook the haddock, turning once, until it is just cooked through, about 5 minutes per side.

5. Remove the fish from the heat and transfer to plates.

6. Serve topped with the cucumber sauce.

INGREDIENT TIP: *There is very little honey in this recipe, about ¼ teaspoon per serving, which equates to about 1.5 grams of carbs. Make sure the honey you use is pure, without added corn syrup or cane sugar, or omit it if you prefer.*

Per Serving Calories: 164; Total Fat: 2g; Cholesterol: 82mg; Sodium: 104mg; Total Carbohydrates: 4g; Sugar: 3g; Fiber: 0g; Protein: 27g

Herb-Crusted Halibut

CARBS PER SERVING: 4G

SERVES 4 / PREP TIME: 10 MINUTES / COOK TIME: 20 MINUTES

The crust on this fish features crushed pistachios, which coat the fish and lock in moisture and flavor. Always use natural pistachios, because the colorful red-dyed ones contain preservatives. You probably also don't want your fillets tinted pink. Pistachios are a great source of protein, antioxidants, vitamin E, and iron. Eating pistachios regularly can help fight cancer, lower cholesterol, and reduce the risk of cardiovascular disease.

4 (5-ounce) halibut fillets
Extra-virgin olive oil,
    for brushing
½ cup coarsely ground
    unsalted pistachios
1 tablespoon chopped
    fresh parsley
1 teaspoon chopped
    fresh thyme
1 teaspoon chopped
    fresh basil
Pinch sea salt
Pinch freshly ground
    black pepper

1. Preheat the oven to 350°F.

2. Line a baking sheet with parchment paper.

3. Pat the halibut fillets dry with a paper towel and place them on the baking sheet.

4. Brush the halibut generously with olive oil.

5. In a small bowl, stir together the pistachios, parsley, thyme, basil, salt, and pepper.

6. Spoon the nut and herb mixture evenly on the fish, spreading it out so the tops of the fillets are covered.

7. Bake the halibut until it flakes when pressed with a fork, about 20 minutes.

8. Serve immediately.

Per Serving Calories: 262; Total Fat: 11g; Cholesterol: 45mg; Sodium: 77mg; Total Carbohydrates: 4g; Sugar: 1g; Fiber: 2g; Protein: 32g

Salmon Florentine

CARBS PER SERVING: 4G

SERVES 4 / PREP TIME: 10 MINUTES / COOK TIME: 30 MINUTES

Salmon is well known for its impressive amount of omega-3 fatty acids. This polyunsaturated fat can reduce the risk of cardiovascular disease and metabolic disease. Salmon can also lower triglycerides, lower blood sugar, and reduce inflammation in the body, which is extremely important for people with type 2 diabetes. You can prepare this dish up to step 6, placing the fish on the greens and keeping it in the refrigerator, covered with aluminum foil, until you are ready to cook the salmon.

1 teaspoon extra-virgin olive oil
½ sweet onion, finely chopped
1 teaspoon minced garlic
3 cups baby spinach
1 cup kale, tough stems removed, torn into 3-inch pieces
Sea salt
Freshly ground black pepper
4 (5-ounce) salmon fillets
Lemon wedges, for serving

1. Preheat the oven to 350°F.

2. Place a large skillet over medium-high heat and add the oil.

3. Sauté the onion and garlic until softened and translucent, about 3 minutes.

4. Add the spinach and kale and sauté until the greens wilt, about 5 minutes.

5. Remove the skillet from the heat and season the greens with salt and pepper.

6. Place the salmon fillets so they are nestled in the greens and partially covered by them. Bake the salmon until it is opaque, about 20 minutes.

7. Serve immediately with a squeeze of fresh lemon.

NUTRITION TIP: *Look for very bright, vibrant spinach leaves, because the paler the color, the less vitamin C these greens contain. Spinach is also a wonderful source of vitamin K, vitamin A, and manganese.*

Per Serving Calories: 281; Total Fat: 16g; Cholesterol: 70mg; Sodium: 91mg; Total Carbohydrates: 4g; Sugar: 1g; Fiber: 1g; Protein: 29g

Baked Salmon with Lemon Sauce

CARBS PER SERVING: 6G

SERVES 4 / PREP TIME: 10 MINUTES / COOK TIME: 15 MINUTES

The lemon sauce in this recipe is great with salmon, and can also be served with chicken or seafood, or spooned over blanched vegetables such as asparagus. The sour cream mellows out the tartness of the lemon, and a touch of honey elevates the sauce to culinary perfection. You might be tempted to just eat it with a spoon rather than serve it for dinner, so make sure you eat dinner right away to avoid the lure.

4 (5-ounce) salmon fillets
Sea salt
Freshly ground black pepper
1 tablespoon extra-virgin olive oil
½ cup low-sodium vegetable broth
Juice and zest of 1 lemon
1 teaspoon chopped fresh thyme
½ cup fat-free sour cream
1 teaspoon honey
1 tablespoon chopped fresh chives

1. Preheat the oven to 400°F.

2. Season the salmon lightly on both sides with salt and pepper.

3. Place a large ovenproof skillet over medium-high heat and add the olive oil.

4. Sear the salmon fillets on both sides until golden, about 3 minutes per side.

5. Transfer the salmon to a baking dish and bake until it is just cooked through, about 10 minutes.

6. While the salmon is baking, whisk together the vegetable broth, lemon juice, zest, and thyme in a small saucepan over medium-high heat until the liquid reduces by about one-quarter, about 5 minutes.

7. Whisk in the sour cream and honey.

8. Stir in the chives and serve the sauce over the salmon.

Per Serving Calories: 310; Total Fat: 18g; Cholesterol: 72mg; Sodium: 129mg; Total Carbohydrates: 6g; Sugar: 2g; Fiber: 0g; Protein: 29g

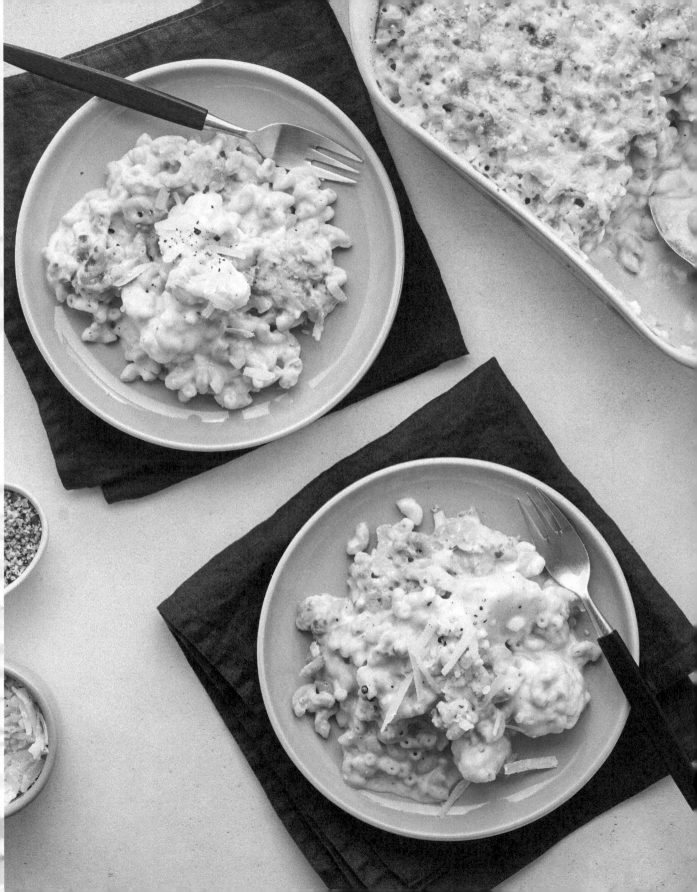

CHAPTER 8

Meatless Mains

Roasted Tomato Bell Pepper Soup

CARBS PER SERVING: 21G

SERVES 6 / PREP TIME: 20 MINUTES / COOK TIME: 35 MINUTES

The scent of roasting garlic will fill your house while you prepare this rich, satisfying soup. Garlic is a time-honored remedy for many health problems, as well as being one of the most popular flavorings worldwide. Garlic is an antioxidant, which means it supports a healthy immune system, and a component in garlic called allicin is very beneficial for people with diabetes. Allicin can help increase the amount of free insulin in the blood, because it competes with insulin for insulin-inactivating sites in the liver. The result is no insulin inactivation by the liver, which means increased amounts of free insulin.

2 tablespoons extra-virgin olive oil, plus more to oil the pan

16 plum tomatoes, cored, halved

4 red bell peppers, seeded, halved

4 celery stalks, coarsely chopped

1 sweet onion, cut into eighths

4 garlic cloves, lightly crushed

Sea salt

Freshly ground black pepper

6 cups low-sodium chicken broth

2 tablespoons chopped fresh basil

2 ounces goat cheese

1. Preheat the oven to 400°F.

2. Lightly oil a large baking dish with olive oil.

3. Place the tomatoes cut-side down in the dish, then scatter the bell peppers, celery, onion, and garlic on the tomatoes.

4. Drizzle the vegetables with 2 tablespoons of olive oil and lightly season with salt and pepper.

5. Roast the vegetables until they are soft and slightly charred, about 30 minutes.

6. Remove the vegetables from the oven and purée them in batches, with the chicken broth, in a food processor or blender until smooth.

7. Transfer the puréed soup to a medium saucepan over medium-high heat and bring the soup to a simmer.

8. Stir in the basil and goat cheese just before serving.

NUTRITION TIP: *Cooked tomatoes are actually healthier for you than raw because the lycopene, an antioxidant found in this fruit, is absorbed more effectively when heated. Yellow and orange tomatoes are also a great source of lycopene.*

Per Serving Calories: 188; Total Fat: 10g; Cholesterol: 10mg; Sodium: 826mg; Total Carbohydrates: 21g; Sugar: 14g; Fiber: 6g; Protein: 8g

Red Lentil Soup

CARBS PER SERVING: 47G

SERVES 8 / PREP TIME: 10 MINUTES / COOK TIME: 55 MINUTES

One of the most satisfying things about lentil soup is the thick texture created by the lentils breaking down during the cooking process, not to mention the chunks of tender carrot and celery visible in the pot and in every spoonful. Carrots are very high in beta-carotene and other more unfamiliar antioxidants such as anthocyanins and hydroxycinnamic acids. Carrots are a powerful weapon against many diseases, including cardiovascular disease and cancer, and they also support good vision.

1 teaspoon extra-virgin olive oil
1 sweet onion, chopped
1 tablespoon minced garlic
4 celery stalks, with the greens, chopped
3 carrots, peeled and diced
3 cups red lentils, picked over, washed, and drained
4 cups low-sodium vegetable broth
3 cups water
2 bay leaves
2 teaspoons chopped fresh thyme
Sea salt
Freshly ground black pepper

1. Place a large stockpot on medium-high heat and add the oil.

2. Sauté the onion and garlic until translucent, about 3 minutes.

3. Stir in the celery and carrots and sauté 5 minutes.

4. Add the lentils, broth, water, and bay leaves, and bring the soup to a boil.

5. Reduce the heat to low and simmer until the lentils are soft and the soup is thick, about 45 minutes.

6. Remove the bay leaves and stir in the thyme.

7. Season with salt and pepper and serve.

Per Serving Calories: 284; Total Fat: 2g; Cholesterol: 0mg; Sodium: 419mg; Total Carbohydrates: 47g; Sugar: 4g; Fiber: 24g; Protein: 20g

Tabbouleh Pita

CARBS PER SERVING: 39G

SERVES 4 / PREP TIME: 20 MINUTES

Tabbouleh is a popular Middle Eastern salad made with tomatoes, parsley, and cooked bulgur wheat or couscous as the base. Stuffing pitas with this complex and colorful mixture is a marvelous way to enjoy the taste and health benefits of all these foods on the go. Make sure you get pitas that are designed for stuffing with hearty fillings, because some products do not open up easily and are better suited for dipping into hummus.

4 whole-wheat pitas
1 cup cooked bulgur wheat
1 English cucumber,
    finely chopped
2 cups halved
    cherry tomatoes
1 yellow bell pepper, seeded
    and finely chopped
2 scallions, white and green
    parts, finely chopped
½ cup finely chopped
    fresh parsley
2 tablespoons extra-virgin
    olive oil
Juice of 1 lemon
Sea salt
Freshly ground black pepper

1. Cut the pitas in half and split them open. Set them aside.

2. In a large bowl, stir together the bulgur, cucumber, tomatoes, bell pepper, scallions, parsley, olive oil, and lemon juice.

3. Season the bulgur mixture with salt and pepper.

4. Spoon the bulgur mixture evenly into the pita halves and serve.

Per Serving Calories: 242; Total Fat: 8g; Cholesterol: 0mg; Sodium: 164mg; Total Carbohydrates: 39g; Sugar: 4g; Fiber: 6g; Protein: 7g

Tomato Baked Beans

CARBS PER SERVING: 48G

SERVES 8 / PREP TIME: 10 MINUTES / COOK TIME: 25 MINUTES

Baked beans are camping and family gathering food: You can imagine them carried in huge iron pots with heavy lids and handles. The beans are often simmered with salt pork, maple syrup, and chile peppers, depending on the geography and the cultural background of the cook. This version of the traditional favorite is a simple, tangy tomato sauce accented with a little Dijon mustard and hot sauce. You can leave the hot sauce out entirely if you want a milder dish.

1 teaspoon extra-virgin
   olive oil
½ sweet onion, chopped
2 teaspoons minced garlic
2 sweet potatoes, peeled
   and diced
1 (28-ounce) can low-sodium
   diced tomatoes
¼ cup sodium-free
   tomato paste
2 tablespoons
   granulated sweetener
2 tablespoons hot sauce
1 tablespoon Dijon mustard
3 (15-ounce) cans sodium-
   free navy or white
   beans, drained
1 tablespoon chopped
   fresh oregano

1. Place a large saucepan over medium-high heat and add the oil.

2. Sauté the onion and garlic until translucent, about 3 minutes.

3. Stir in the sweet potatoes, diced tomatoes, tomato paste, sweetener, hot sauce, and mustard and bring to a boil.

4. Reduce the heat and simmer the tomato sauce for 10 minutes.

5. Stir in the beans and simmer for 10 minutes more.

6. Stir in the oregano and serve.

Per Serving Calories: 255; Total Fat: 2g; Cholesterol: 0mg; Sodium: 149mg; Total Carbohydrates: 48g; Sugar: 8g; Fiber: 12g; Protein: 15g

Vegetarian Three-Bean Chili

CARBS PER SERVING: 45G

SERVES 8 / PREP TIME: 20 MINUTES / COOK TIME: 1 HOUR

There is a great deal going on in this chili. Every spoonful is bursting with beans, tomatoes, spices, and vegetables. This recipe makes more than enough for dinner leftovers the next day or lunches for two days. You can also scoop this chili onto homemade whole-grain tortilla chips for a filling snack.

1 teaspoon extra-virgin olive oil

1 sweet onion, chopped

1 red bell pepper, seeded and diced

1 green bell pepper, seeded and diced

2 teaspoons minced garlic

1 (28-ounce) can low-sodium diced tomatoes

1 (15-ounce) can sodium-free black beans, rinsed and drained

1 (15-ounce) can sodium-free red kidney beans, rinsed and drained

1 (15-ounce) can sodium-free navy beans, rinsed and drained

2 tablespoons chili powder

2 teaspoons ground cumin

1 teaspoon ground coriander

¼ teaspoon red pepper flakes

1. Place a large saucepan over medium-high heat and add the oil.

2. Sauté the onion, red and green bell peppers, and garlic until the vegetables have softened, about 5 minutes.

3. Add the tomatoes, black beans, red kidney beans, navy beans, chili powder, cumin, coriander, and red pepper flakes to the pan.

4. Bring the chili to a boil, then reduce the heat to low.

5. Simmer the chili, stirring occasionally, for at least 1 hour.

6. Serve hot.

COOKING TIP: *Chili tastes best the next day, after the spices have had time to mellow and deepen in flavor, so whenever possible, make this recipe the day before you want to serve it.*

Per Serving Calories: 479; Total Fat: 28g; Cholesterol: 0mg; Sodium: 15mg; Total Carbohydrates: 45g; Sugar: 4g; Fiber: 17g; Protein: 15g

Chickpea Lentil Curry

CARBS PER SERVING: 50G

SERVES 6 / PREP TIME: 10 MINUTES / COOK TIME: 25 MINUTES

Lentils should be part of any diet, unless you have an allergy or sensitivity, because they are a stellar source of fiber; low in fat and calories; and high in B vitamins, protein, and iron. This legume is the whole nutrition package—and it's inexpensive as well. Lentils can help stabilize blood sugar, boost energy, support digestive and cardiovascular health, and lower cholesterol. You can either cook your own lentils for this dish or buy a low-sodium canned product.

1 tablespoon extra-virgin olive oil

1 sweet onion, chopped

1 tablespoon grated fresh ginger

1 teaspoon minced garlic

2 tablespoons red curry paste

1 teaspoon ground cumin

½ teaspoon turmeric

Pinch cayenne pepper

1 (28-ounce) can sodium-free diced tomatoes

2 cups cooked lentils

1 (15-ounce) can water-packed chickpeas, rinsed and drained

¼ cup coconut milk

2 tablespoons chopped fresh cilantro

1. Place a large saucepan over medium-high heat and add the oil.

2. Sauté the onion, ginger, and garlic until softened, about 3 minutes.

3. Add the curry paste, cumin, turmeric, and cayenne and sauté 1 minute more.

4. Stir in the tomatoes, lentils, chickpeas, and coconut milk.

5. Bring the curry to a boil, then reduce the heat to low and simmer for 20 minutes.

6. Remove the curry from the heat and garnish with the cilantro.

NUTRITION TIP: *Chickpeas, also known as garbanzo beans, are prized for their fiber content, which can help lower cholesterol levels. Garbanzo beans also improve blood sugar levels and help control insulin secretion.*

Per Serving Calories: 338; Total Fat: 8g; Cholesterol: 0mg; Sodium: 22mg; Total Carbohydrates: 50g; Sugar: 9g; Fiber: 20g; Protein: 18g

Ricotta Quinoa Bake

CARBS PER SERVING: 38G

SERVES 4 / PREP TIME: 20 MINUTES / COOK TIME: 30 MINUTES

Ricotta adds a wonderfully tangy flavor and slightly grainy texture to this comforting casserole. If you prefer cottage cheese, that's a fine substitute, but there are some differences between the two. Ricotta is produced from the whey that is left over after making other cheeses, such as mozzarella, and cottage cheese is made from coagulated milk. Ricotta is significantly lower in sodium than cottage cheese, so it's also a great choice for anyone watching their blood pressure.

1 teaspoon extra-virgin olive oil
½ sweet onion, chopped
2 teaspoons minced garlic
2 cups cooked quinoa
2 eggs
½ cup low-fat ricotta cheese
Sea salt
Freshly ground black pepper
2 cups cherry tomatoes
1 zucchini, cut into thin ribbons
⅛ cup pine nuts, toasted

1. Preheat the oven to 350°F.

2. Place a medium skillet over medium-high heat and add the olive oil.

3. Sauté the onion and garlic until softened and translucent, about 3 minutes.

4. Remove the skillet from the heat and stir in the quinoa, eggs, and ricotta.

5. Season the mixture with salt and pepper.

6. Stir in the cherry tomatoes and spoon the casserole into an 8-by-8-inch baking dish.

7. Scatter the zucchini ribbons and pine nuts on top, and bake the casserole until it is heated through, about 25 minutes.

Per Serving Calories: 302; Total Fat: 9g; Cholesterol: 120mg; Sodium: 234mg; Total Carbohydrates: 38g; Sugar: 5g; Fiber: 4g; Protein: 17g

Creamy Mac and Cheese

CARBS PER SERVING: 44G

SERVES 6 / PREP TIME: 10 MINUTES / COOK TIME: 25 MINUTES

Mac and cheese is the ultimate cuddling on the couch in your fuzzy slippers and robe food. Comfort oozes out of each spoonful, along with a generous amount of delicious cheese sauce made with three kinds of cheese! The evaporated milk and low-fat cheeses keep the calories and fat in this dish in the low range, so feel no guilt when you dig in and enjoy. Other kinds of pasta can be tossed in this sauce, if you're out of the traditional elbow noodles.

1 cup fat-free evaporated milk
½ cup skim milk
½ cup low-fat cottage cheese
½ cup low-fat Cheddar cheese
1 teaspoon nutmeg
Pinch cayenne pepper
Sea salt
Freshly ground black pepper
6 cups cooked whole-wheat
    elbow macaroni
2 tablespoons grated
    Parmesan cheese

1. Preheat the oven to 350°F.

2. Place a large saucepan over low heat and add the evaporated milk and skim milk.

3. Heat the evaporated milk and skim milk until steaming, then stir in the cottage cheese and Cheddar, stirring until they melt.

4. Stir in the nutmeg and cayenne.

5. Season the sauce with salt and black pepper and remove from the heat.

6. Stir the cooked pasta into the sauce, then spoon the mac and cheese into a large casserole dish.

7. Sprinkle the top with the Parmesan cheese, and bake until it is bubbly and lightly browned, about 20 minutes.

Per Serving Calories: 246; Total Fat: 2g; Cholesterol: 6mg; Sodium: 187mg; Total Carbohydrates: 44g; Sugar: 7g; Fiber: 4g; Protein: 16g

Spaghetti Puttanesca

CARBS PER SERVING: 35G

SERVES 6 / PREP TIME: 20 MINUTES / COOK TIME: 35 MINUTES

Tomatoes are a little like apples; you should eat at least one a day for optimal health. If you don't want to bite into your daily tomato like a crisp apple, this spicy sauce will certainly give you the recommended amount. Tomatoes are high in potassium, vitamin B_6, niacin, folate, and antioxidants such as carotenoids. Tomatoes are heart-friendly, reduce hypertension, and can lower both cholesterol and your risk of cancer.

1 tablespoon extra-virgin olive oil

1 sweet onion, chopped

2 celery stalks, chopped

3 teaspoons minced garlic

2 (28-ounce) cans sodium-free diced tomatoes

2 tablespoons chopped fresh basil

1 tablespoon chopped fresh oregano

½ teaspoon red pepper flakes

½ cup quartered, pitted Kalamata olives

¼ cup freshly squeezed lemon juice

8 ounces whole-wheat spaghetti

1. Place a large saucepan over medium-high heat and add the oil.

2. Sauté the onion, celery, and garlic until they are translucent, about 3 minutes.

3. Add the tomatoes, basil, oregano, and red pepper flakes, and bring the sauce to a boil, stirring occasionally.

4. Reduce the heat to low and simmer 20 minutes, stirring occasionally.

5. Stir in the olives and lemon juice and remove the saucepan from the heat.

6. Cook the pasta according to the package instructions.

7. Spoon the sauce over the pasta and serve.

INGREDIENT TIP: *Kalamata olives are one of the most sought-after type of this fruit because of their deep and complex flavor. Do not just use ordinary black olives; look for the real thing, even if you have to pit them.*

Per Serving Calories: 200; Total Fat: 5g; Cholesterol: 28mg; Sodium: 88mg; Total Carbohydrates: 35g; Sugar: 8g; Fiber: 4g; Protein: 7g

Vegetable Kale Lasagna

CARBS PER SERVING: 48G

SERVES 6 / PREP TIME: 20 MINUTES / COOK TIME: 1 HOUR

Lasagna can be a lot of work—all that cooking and layering of the fillings—but the end result is well worth the effort. Plus you will have leftovers. If you prefer fresh pasta, use six sheets to form three layers. Most supermarkets carry fresh whole-wheat lasagna sheets in their produce or specialty sections. Spinach or sun-dried tomato noodles would also be appealing in this dish.

1 tablespoon extra-virgin olive oil

1 sweet onion, chopped

2 teaspoons minced garlic

½ small eggplant, chopped

1 green zucchini, chopped

1 yellow zucchini, chopped

1 red bell pepper, seeded and diced

1 (28-ounce) can sodium-free diced tomatoes

1 cup shredded kale

1 tablespoon chopped fresh basil

2 teaspoons chopped fresh oregano

Pinch red pepper flakes

12 whole-wheat lasagna noodles, cooked according to package instructions

½ cup grated Parmesan cheese

½ cup fat-free mozzarella cheese

1. Preheat the oven to 400°F.

2. Place a large saucepan over medium-high heat and add the olive oil.

3. Sauté the onion and garlic until softened and translucent, about 3 minutes.

4. Stir in the eggplant, green and yellow zucchini, bell pepper, tomatoes, and kale.

5. Bring the sauce to a boil, then reduce the heat to low and simmer for 15 minutes.

6. Remove the sauce from the heat and stir in the basil, oregano, and red pepper flakes.

7. Scoop one quarter of the sauce into a 9-by-13-inch rectangular baking pan. Top with 4 noodles. Repeat with a layer of sauce, noodles, sauce, noodles, and the final layer of sauce on top. Sprinkle with the Parmesan cheese and mozzarella.

8. Bake the lasagna until it's bubbly and hot, about 45 minutes.

9. Cool for 10 minutes and serve.

Per Serving Calories: 313; Total Fat: 8g; Cholesterol: 32mg; Sodium: 165mg; Total Carbohydrates: 48g; Sugar: 7g; Fiber: 5g; Protein: 16g

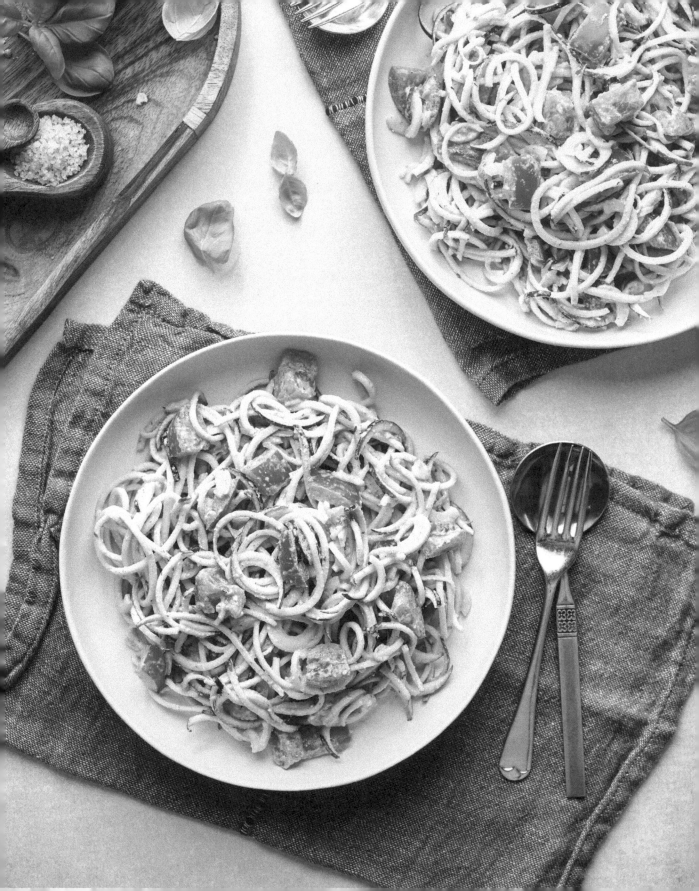

CHAPTER 9

Vegetable Sides

Nutmeg Green Beans

CARBS PER SERVING: 12G

SERVES 4 / PREP TIME: 15 MINUTES / COOK TIME: 5 MINUTES

Simple in preparation but wonderfully complex in taste, green beans become a little exotic and almost rich when tossed in butter and nutmeg. If you grate your own nutmeg, using a micrograter on a whole nutmeg seed kernel, you will be amazed at the strength of flavor of this unassuming spice. Whole nutmeg can be found in the spice section of some supermarkets, and you can store it in a sealed container along with the little grater for up to one month.

1 tablespoon butter
1½ pounds green
    beans, trimmed
1 teaspoon ground nutmeg
Sea salt

1. Place a large skillet over medium heat and melt the butter.

2. Add the green beans and sauté, stirring often, until the beans are tender-crisp, about 5 minutes.

3. Stir in the nutmeg and season with salt.

4. Serve immediately.

NUTRITION TIP: *Green beans, or string beans, are packed with antioxidants, vitamin K, manganese, and fiber. Green beans are very heart-friendly and boost the immune system.*

Per Serving Calories: 81; Total Fat: 3g; Cholesterol: 8mg; Sodium: 89mg; Total Carbohydrates: 12g; Sugar: 3g; Fiber: 6g; Protein: 3g

Golden Lemony Wax Beans

CARBS PER SERVING: 8G

SERVES 4 / PREP TIME: 5 MINUTES / COOK TIME: 15 MINUTES

Wax beans are the pretty pale yellow beans that some people call yellow green beans. Wax beans are stringless and often have pale green legumes in their slightly matte yellow shells. They are low in calories, about 40 per cup, and contain a hearty dose of dietary fiber, about 4 grams per cup. Look for young, tender beans with a satisfying snap for a succulent taste.

2 pounds wax beans

2 tablespoons extra-virgin olive oil

Sea salt

Freshly ground black pepper

Juice of ½ lemon

1. Preheat the oven to 400°F.

2. Line a baking sheet with aluminum foil.

3. In a large bowl, toss the beans and olive oil. Season lightly with salt and pepper.

4. Transfer the beans to the baking sheet and spread them out.

5. Roast the beans until caramelized and tender, about 10 to 12 minutes.

6. Transfer the beans to a serving platter and sprinkle with the lemon juice.

Per Serving Calories: 100; Total Fat: 7g; Cholesterol: 0mg; Sodium: 813mg; Total Carbohydrates: 8g; Sugar: 4g; Fiber: 4g; Protein: 2g

Broiled Spinach

CARBS PER SERVING: 2G

SERVES 4 / PREP TIME: 5 MINUTES / COOK TIME: 4 MINUTES

You might think broiling dark leafy greens would create a mushy mess, but this recipe produces incredible crispy spinach that is a perfect side dish for robust meats. The trick is to make sure the spinach is completely coated with oil so that each piece crisps up, and to spread the spinach out evenly on the rack, with almost no overlap. You can use any seasonings you like, such as coriander, paprika, or cayenne, for different variations.

8 cups spinach, thoroughly washed and spun dry
1 tablespoon extra-virgin olive oil
¼ teaspoon ground cumin
Sea salt
Freshly ground black pepper

1. Preheat the broiler. Put an oven rack in the upper third of the oven.

2. Set a wire rack on a large baking sheet.

3. In a large bowl, massage the spinach, oil, and cumin together until all the leaves are well coated.

4. Spread half the spinach out on the rack, with as little overlap as possible. Season the greens lightly with salt and pepper.

5. Broil the spinach until the edges are crispy, about 2 minutes.

6. Remove the baking sheet from the oven and transfer the spinach to a large serving bowl.

7. Repeat with the remaining spinach.

8. Serve immediately.

Per Serving Calories: 40; Total Fat: 4g; Cholesterol: 0mg; Sodium: 106mg; Total Carbohydrates: 2g; Sugar: 0g; Fiber: 1g; Protein: 2g

Wilted Kale and Chard

CARBS PER SERVING: 16G

SERVES 4 / PREP TIME: 10 MINUTES / COOK TIME: 10 MINUTES

Wilted greens might not sound like the most appealing dish, but it's actually bursting with flavor, and looks gorgeous next to dishes like mashed sweet potato and snowy baked halibut. Don't wilt the greens so much that they lose their texture and become a mushy mess; just toss until they are tender but still hold their shape. Cardamom adds a delicate citrus taste to the greens that is mirrored by the fresh lemon juice.

2 tablespoons extra-virgin olive oil

1 pound kale, coarse stems removed and leaves chopped

1 pound Swiss chard, coarse stems removed and leaves chopped

1 tablespoon freshly squeezed lemon juice

½ teaspoon ground cardamom

Sea salt

Freshly ground black pepper

1. Place a large skillet over medium-high heat and add the olive oil.

2. Add the kale, chard, lemon juice, and cardamom to the skillet. Use tongs to toss the greens continuously until they are wilted, about 10 minutes or less.

3. Season the greens with salt and pepper.

4. Serve immediately.

Per Serving Calories: 140; Total Fat: 7g; Cholesterol: 0mg; Sodium: 351mg; Total Carbohydrates: 16g; Sugar: 1g; Fiber: 4g; Protein: 6g

Sautéed Garlicky Mushrooms

CARBS PER SERVING: 8G

SERVES 4 / PREP TIME: 10 MINUTES / COOK TIME: 12 MINUTES

Mushrooms have a satisfying meaty texture, and they easily soak up flavors such as garlic and herbs. Button or white mushrooms are usually inexpensive and a good size for sautéing as a side. You can certainly try what might be considered higher-end fungi, such as cremini, shiitake, or baby portobellas, for a different look and flavor. This simple side would be lovely with a grilled steak or roasted pork tenderloin.

1 tablespoon butter

2 teaspoons extra-virgin olive oil

2 pounds button mushrooms, halved

2 teaspoons minced fresh garlic

1 teaspoon chopped fresh thyme

Sea salt

Freshly ground black pepper

1. Place a large skillet over medium-high heat and add the butter and olive oil.

2. Sauté the mushrooms, stirring occasionally, until they are lightly caramelized and tender, about 10 minutes.

3. Add the garlic and thyme and sauté for 2 more minutes.

4. Season the mushrooms with salt and pepper before serving.

INGREDIENT TIP: *The way you store your mushrooms can negatively affect the phytonutrient content. Never store them at room temperature: 38°F is ideal.*

Per Serving Calories: 97; Total Fat: 6g; Cholesterol: 8mg; Sodium: 92mg; Total Carbohydrates: 8g; Sugar: 4g; Fiber: 2g; Protein: 7g

Sesame Bok Choy with Almonds

CARBS PER SERVING: 8G

SERVES 4 / PREP TIME: 15 MINUTES / COOK TIME: 7 MINUTES

Bok choy is an elegant vegetable often used in Asian cuisines. Look for baby bok choy for this dish, and spend some time cleaning the dirt out of the spaces between the stalks at the base. Bok choy contains over 70 antioxidants, impressive amounts of vitamin A, C, and K, as well as potassium, calcium, and iron. The anti-inflammatory benefits of bok choy alone make it a highly desirable choice for a type 2 diabetes diet—or any diet, for that matter.

2 teaspoons sesame oil
2 pounds bok choy, cleaned and quartered
2 teaspoons low-sodium soy sauce
Pinch red pepper flakes
½ cup toasted sliced almonds

1. Place a large skillet over medium heat and add the oil.

2. When the oil is hot, sauté the bok choy until tender-crisp, about 5 minutes.

3. Stir in the soy sauce and red pepper flakes and sauté 2 minutes more.

4. Remove the bok choy to a serving bowl and top with the sliced almonds.

SUBSTITUTION TIP: *Toasted sesame seeds can be a lovely substitution for the almonds, if you want to double up on the rich sesame flavor. Use about 2 tablespoons of seeds.*

Per Serving Calories: 119; Total Fat: 8g; Cholesterol: 0mg; Sodium: 294mg; Total Carbohydrates: 8g; Sugar: 3g; Fiber: 4g; Protein: 6g

Asparagus with Cashews

CARBS PER SERVING: 14G

SERVES 4 / PREP TIME: 10 MINUTES / COOK TIME: 20 MINUTES

Asparagus seems like it would be too delicate to cook well on a grill or roasted in a very hot oven, but it caramelizes easily and holds up beautifully. The creamy, crunchy texture of the cashews accents this vegetable perfectly. Cashews are very high in copper and are a good source of phosphorus, manganese, and zinc. You can also use hazelnuts or pistachios. Just make sure you get unsalted nuts, with no colors or flavors added.

2 pounds asparagus, woody ends trimmed
1 tablespoon extra-virgin olive oil
Sea salt
Freshly ground black pepper
½ cup chopped cashews
Zest and juice of 1 lime

1. Preheat the oven to 400°F and line a baking sheet with aluminum foil.

2. In a large bowl, toss the asparagus with the oil and lightly season with salt and pepper.

3. Transfer the asparagus to the baking sheet and bake until tender and lightly browned, 15 to 20 minutes.

4. Transfer the asparagus to a serving bowl and toss them with the chopped cashews, lime zest, and lime juice.

Per Serving Calories: 174; Total Fat: 12g; Cholesterol: 0mg; Sodium: 66mg; Total Carbohydrates: 14g; Sugar: 5g; Fiber: 5g; Protein: 8g

Horseradish Mashed Cauliflower

CARBS PER SERVING: 20G

SERVES 4 / PREP TIME: 5 MINUTES / COOK TIME: 10 MINUTES

Mashed cauliflower is so close in texture to mashed potatoes that your family might not notice the difference, especially when the mash is heavily spiked with hot horseradish. You can also try roasted garlic, sweet butter, goat cheese, and chopped scallions in your mash—pretty much anything you would mix with potatoes. Make sure you drain your cooked cauliflower very well before mashing it, or you will end up with a watery rather than a fluffy dish.

1 large head cauliflower (about 3 pounds), cut into small florets

½ cup skim milk

2 tablespoons prepared horseradish

¼ teaspoon sea salt

2 teaspoons chopped fresh chives

1. Place a large pot of water on high heat and bring it to a boil.

2. Blanch the cauliflower until it is tender, about 5 minutes.

3. Drain the cauliflower completely and transfer it to a food processor.

4. Add the milk and horseradish to the cauliflower and purée until it is smooth and thick, about 2 minutes. Or mash it by hand with a potato masher.

5. Transfer the mashed cauliflower to a bowl and season with salt.

6. Serve immediately, topped with the chopped chives.

INGREDIENT TIP: *Whole horseradish root is sometimes available in the produce section, so you can make your own. Peel fresh horseradish and then grate it. Add it to the mashed cauliflower a little at a time, as it can be very strong, until you have the desired flavor.*

Per Serving Calories: 100; Total Fat: 0g; Cholesterol: 1mg; Sodium: 259mg; Total Carbohydrates: 20g; Sugar: 10g; Fiber: 9g; Protein: 8g

Broccoli Cauliflower Bake

CARBS PER SERVING: 14G

SERVES 6 / PREP TIME: 15 MINUTES / COOK TIME: 40 MINUTES

Casserole side dishes can seem so decadent, especially when cheese sauce is involved. This one certainly tastes decadent, but it's easy to put together. Then simply pop the casserole dish in the oven and you're free to whip up whatever else you are having with your meal.

½ cup ground almonds
¼ cup grated
   Parmesan cheese
1 tablespoon butter, melted,
   plus 2 tablespoons butter
Pinch freshly ground
   black pepper
1 head broccoli, cut into
   small florets
1 head cauliflower, cut into
   small florets
1 sweet onion, chopped
1 teaspoon minced garlic
2 tablespoons all-
   purpose flour
1 cup skim milk
2 ounces goat cheese
¼ teaspoon ground nutmeg

1. Preheat the oven to 350°F.

2. In a small bowl, mix together the almonds, Parmesan cheese, melted butter, and pepper. Set it aside.

3. Place a large pot full of water over high heat and bring to a boil.

4. Blanch the broccoli and cauliflower for 1 minute, drain, and set them aside.

5. Place a large skillet over medium-high heat and melt the 2 tablespoons of butter.

6. Sauté the onion and garlic until tender, about 3 minutes. Whisk in the flour and cook, stirring constantly, for 1 minute. Whisk in the milk and cook, stirring constantly, until the sauce has thickened, about 4 minutes.

7. Remove the skillet from the heat and whisk in the goat cheese and nutmeg.

8. Add the broccoli and cauliflower, then spoon the mixture into a 1½-quart casserole dish.

9. Sprinkle the almond mixture over the top and bake until the casserole is heated through, about 30 minutes.

COOKING TIP: *If you need a make-ahead casserole for a family event or a potluck dinner, this is a wonderful choice. Put it together completely through step 8 (including topping with the almond mixture), and just bake it right from the refrigerator for 45 minutes.*

Per Serving Calories: 224; Total Fat: 7g; Cholesterol: 29mg; Sodium: 178mg; Total Carbohydrates: 14g; Sugar: 6g; Fiber: 5g; Protein: 11g

Ginger Broccoli

CARBS PER SERVING: 14G

SERVES 4 / PREP TIME: 10 MINUTES / COOK TIME: 10 MINUTES

Ginger and broccoli spend a great deal of time together, because the florets soak up the heat of the spice and create magic. The Asian varieties of broccoli are a key ingredient in Asian cooking, where ginger marries with soy sauce and garlic in many dishes. Serve this dish alongside a less assertively spiced main course, so that you can enjoy the diversity rather than being inundated with too many flavors.

1 tablespoon extra-virgin olive oil
½ sweet onion, thinly sliced
2 teaspoons grated fresh ginger
1 teaspoon minced fresh garlic
2 heads broccoli, cut into small florets
¼ cup low-sodium chicken broth
Sea salt
Freshly ground black pepper

1. Place a large skillet over medium-high heat and add the oil.

2. Sauté the onion, ginger, and garlic until softened, about 3 minutes.

3. Add the broccoli florets and chicken broth, and sauté until the broccoli is tender, about 5 minutes.

4. Season with salt and pepper.

5. Serve immediately.

Per Serving Calories: 102; Total Fat: 4g; Cholesterol: 0mg; Sodium: 109mg; Total Carbohydrates: 14g; Sugar: 4g; Fiber: 5g; Protein: 5g

Sautéed Mixed Vegetables

CARBS PER SERVING: 18G

SERVES 4 / PREP TIME: 20 MINUTES / COOK TIME: 8 MINUTES

Fine restaurants create culinary art using the colors of various vegetables either as a backdrop or as the central focus of the plate. A main course, even a plain roasted chicken breast, can look spectacular beside a vibrant rainbow of vegetables, especially when they have all sorts of shapes and textures. To perk up the flavor of this beautiful dish, swap a teaspoon of butter for 1 teaspoon of the olive oil.

2 teaspoons extra-virgin olive oil
2 carrots, peeled and sliced
4 cups broccoli florets
4 cups cauliflower florets
1 red bell pepper, seeded and cut into long strips
1 cup green beans, trimmed
Sea salt
Freshly ground black pepper

1. Place a large skillet over medium heat and add the olive oil.

2. Sauté the carrots, broccoli, and cauliflower until tender-crisp, about 6 minutes.

3. Add the bell pepper and green beans, and sauté 2 minutes more.

4. Season with salt and pepper, and serve.

SUBSTITUTION TIP: *The vegetables listed here are just a suggestion. Use whatever you have in the refrigerator, or the freshest choice from the market. Get an assortment of colors so the dish is visually pleasing.*

Per Serving Calories: 106; Total Fat: 3g; Cholesterol: 0mg; Sodium: 142mg; Total Carbohydrates: 18g; Sugar: 7g; Fiber: 7g; Protein: 6g

Zucchini Noodles with Lime-Basil Pesto

CARBS PER SERVING: 10G

SERVES 4 / PREP TIME: 20 MINUTES

Spring on a plate pretty much describes the mélange of greens and creams that make up this delicate side dish. If you have never used a spiralizer, once you start you might find yourself creating curly noodles out of everything in your kitchen. Zucchini works particularly well because it has the right texture to mimic real cooked noodles, and the vegetable is round enough to create strands of incredible length. Both yellow and green zucchini are great choices.

2 cups packed fresh
    basil leaves
½ cup pine nuts
2 teaspoons minced garlic
Zest and juice of 1 lime
Pinch sea salt
Pinch freshly ground
    black pepper
¼ cup extra-virgin olive oil
4 green or yellow zucchini,
    rinsed, dried, and julienned
    or spiralized
1 tomato, diced

1. Place the basil, pine nuts, garlic, lime zest, lime juice, salt, and pepper in a food processor or a blender and pulse until very finely chopped.

2. While the machine is running, add the olive oil in a thin stream until a thick paste forms.

3. In a large bowl, combine the zucchini noodles and tomato. Add the pesto by the tablespoonful until you have the desired flavor. Serve the zucchini pasta immediately.

4. Store any leftover pesto in a sealed container in the refrigerator for up to 2 weeks.

SUBSTITUTION TIP: *You can spiralize a broad range of produce, from zucchini to carrots to apples. Feel free to experiment with ingredients other than zucchini for a unique side dish.*

Per Serving Calories: 261; Total Fat: 23g; Cholesterol: 0mg; Sodium: 80mg; Total Carbohydrates: 10g; Sugar: 5g; Fiber: 3g; Protein: 5g

Spaghetti Squash with Sun-Dried Tomatoes

CARBS PER SERVING: 13G

SERVES 4 / PREP TIME: 20 MINUTES / COOK TIME: 1 HOUR, 10 MINUTES

Pale yellow squash, flecks of bright red, green accents, and a scattering of crunchy golden sunflower seeds create a tantalizing visual feast. Sprinkle some feta cheese or goat cheese on top for a little extra protein if you plan to eat the dish as a dinner or a filling lunch on its own.

1 spaghetti squash, halved and seeded

3 teaspoons extra-virgin olive oil, divided

¼ sweet onion, chopped

1 teaspoon minced garlic

2 cups fresh spinach

¼ cup chopped sun-dried tomatoes

¼ cup roasted, shelled sunflower seeds

Juice of ½ lemon

Sea salt

Freshly ground black pepper

1. Preheat the oven to 350°F. Line a baking sheet with parchment paper.

2. Place the squash on the baking sheet and brush the cut edges with 2 teaspoons of olive oil.

3. Bake the squash until it is tender and separates into strands with a fork, about 1 hour.

4. Let the squash cool for 5 minutes then use a fork to scrape out the strands from both halves of the squash. Cover the squash strands and set them aside.

5. Place a large skillet over medium-high heat and add the remaining 1 teaspoon of olive oil. Sauté the onion and garlic until softened and translucent, about 3 minutes.

6. Stir in the spinach and sun-dried tomatoes, and sauté until the spinach is wilted, about 4 minutes.

7. Remove the skillet from the heat and stir in the squash strands, sunflower seeds, and lemon juice.

8. Season with salt and pepper and serve warm.

COOKING TIP: *Spaghetti squash can be cooked ahead of time. Scrape strands into a container and store in the refrigerator for up to 2 days. Let it sit at room temperature for 15 minutes, then add it to the skillet right after the onion and garlic in step 5. Stir until heated through, about 6 minutes, and continue with the recipe as directed.*

Per Serving Calories: 103; Total Fat: 6g; Cholesterol: 0mg; Sodium: 163mg; Total Carbohydrates: 13g; Sugar: 2g; Fiber: 1g; Protein: 3g

Sun-Dried Tomato Brussels Sprouts

CARBS PER SERVING: 14G

SERVES 4 / PREP TIME: 15 MINUTES / COOK TIME: 20 MINUTES

Brussels sprouts are a member of the cruciferous vegetable family, along with cauliflower and cabbage, which is easy to see because these adorable sprouts look like mini cabbages. Like the other vegetables in this group, Brussels sprouts can help lower cholesterol, prevent cancer, and support healthy thyroid function.

1 pound Brussels sprouts, trimmed and halved
1 tablespoon extra-virgin olive oil
Sea salt
Freshly ground black pepper
½ cup sun-dried tomatoes, chopped
2 tablespoons freshly squeezed lemon juice
1 teaspoon lemon zest

1. Preheat the oven to 400°F. Line a large baking sheet with aluminum foil.

2. In a large bowl, toss the Brussels sprouts with oil and season with salt and pepper.

3. Spread the Brussels sprouts on the baking sheet in a single layer.

4. Roast the sprouts until they are caramelized, about 20 minutes.

5. Transfer the sprouts to a serving bowl. Mix in the sun-dried tomatoes, lemon juice, and lemon zest.

6. Stir to combine, and serve.

INGREDIENT TIP: *Take care to not overcook Brussels sprouts because doing so will reduce their nutritional value and produce an unpleasant taste and smell.*

Per Serving Calories: 110; Total Fat: 6g; Cholesterol: 0mg; Sodium: 105mg; Total Carbohydrates: 14g; Sugar: 3g; Fiber: 5g; Protein: 5g

Pico de Gallo Navy Beans

CARBS PER SERVING: 34G

SERVES 4 / PREP TIME: 20 MINUTES

Pico de Gallo is an uncooked salsa that features the colors of the Mexican flag—green, white, and red—so is also called *salsa bandera* (flag salsa). This fresh salsa is often served with refried beans or as a filling for corn tacos, but it also works well as a side dish. The cooked navy beans are a mellow counterpoint to the spices and hot pepper. Try this side with grilled chicken or as a topping on a piece of baked salmon or tilapia.

2½ cups cooked navy beans
1 tomato, diced
½ red bell pepper, seeded and chopped
¼ jalapeño pepper, chopped
1 scallion, white and green parts, chopped
1 teaspoon minced garlic
1 teaspoon ground cumin
½ teaspoon ground coriander
½ cup low-sodium feta cheese

1. Put the beans, tomato, bell pepper, jalapeño, scallion, garlic, cumin, and coriander in a medium bowl and stir until well mixed.

2. Top with the feta cheese and serve.

Per Serving Calories: 224; Total Fat: 4g; Cholesterol: 13mg; Sodium: 164mg; Total Carbohydrates: 34g; Sugar: 4g; Fiber: 13g; Protein: 14g

Fennel and Chickpeas

CARBS PER SERVING: 32G

SERVES 6 / PREP TIME: 10 MINUTES / COOK TIME: 20 MINUTES

Fennel might be an unfamiliar vegetable to you, but its subtle licorice flavor and crunchy texture will win you over after the first bite. It is often found in Mediterranean cooking. The bulbous vegetable is related to carrots and parsley and is an excellent source of vitamin C, fiber, potassium, and manganese. Fennel is also packed with antioxidants, so it provides immune system support and promotes healthy cardiovascular and digestive systems.

1 tablespoon extra-virgin olive oil

1 small fennel bulb, trimmed and cut into ¼-inch-thick slices

1 sweet onion, thinly sliced

1 (15½-ounce) can sodium-free chickpeas, rinsed and drained

1 cup low-sodium chicken broth

2 teaspoons chopped fresh thyme

¼ teaspoon sea salt

¼ teaspoon freshly ground black pepper

1 tablespoon butter

1. Place a large saucepan over medium-high heat and add the oil.

2. Sauté the fennel and onion until tender and lightly browned, about 10 minutes.

3. Add the chickpeas, broth, thyme, salt, and pepper.

4. Cover and cook, stirring occasionally, for 10 minutes, until the liquid has reduced by about half.

5. Remove the pan from the heat and stir in the butter.

6. Serve hot.

Per Serving Calories: 215; Total Fat: 5g; Cholesterol: 5mg; Sodium: 253mg; Total Carbohydrates: 32g; Sugar: 2g; Fiber: 15g; Protein: 12g

Italian Roasted Vegetables

CARBS PER SERVING: 11G

SERVES 4 / PREP TIME: 15 MINUTES / COOK TIME: 20 MINUTES

Roasted vegetables can be found in many cuisines, as vegetables tend to be inexpensive and the preparation is simple. Roasting allows the taste of the individual vegetables to shine through, because there is no camouflaging sauce. Watch the cherry tomatoes when you serve this side, because when they are cooked this way, they can explode when punctured with a fork. Let the vegetables sit for a couple of minutes to allow the tomatoes to deflate a little.

2 tablespoons extra-virgin olive oil

2 teaspoons chopped fresh oregano

1 teaspoon chopped fresh basil

1 teaspoon minced garlic

½ pound whole cremini mushrooms

2 cups cauliflower florets

1 zucchini, cut into 1-inch chunks

2 cups cherry tomatoes

Sea salt

Freshly ground black pepper

1. Preheat the oven to 400°F. Line a baking sheet with aluminum foil.

2. In a large bowl, stir together the oil, oregano, basil, and garlic.

3. Add the mushrooms, cauliflower, zucchini, and cherry tomatoes and toss to coat.

4. Transfer the vegetables to the baking sheet and roast until they are tender and lightly browned, about 20 minutes.

5. Season with salt and pepper and serve.

Per Serving Calories: 115; Total Fat: 8g; Cholesterol: 0mg; Sodium: 86mg; Total Carbohydrates: 11g; Sugar: 5g; Fiber: 4g; Protein: 4g

Roasted Eggplant with Goat Cheese

CARBS PER SERVING: 7G

SERVES 4 / PREP TIME: 15 MINUTES / COOK TIME: 20 MINUTES

This recipe is relatively low in carbs, which is surprising considering that eggplant is mainly a carbohydrate. This shiny vegetable sucks up fat like a sponge because of its texture, so be careful how much oil you use when cooking it. Eggplant is a great source of vitamin A, vitamin C, potassium, niacin, and antioxidants, making it heart healthy and an excellent choice to cut your risk of cancer.

1 pound eggplant, cut into 1-inch chunks
2 tablespoons extra-virgin olive oil
Sea salt
Freshly ground black pepper
2 tablespoons balsamic vinegar
2 ounces goat cheese, crumbled
2 teaspoons chopped fresh basil

1. Preheat the oven to 400°F. Line a baking sheet with aluminum foil.

2. In a large bowl, toss the eggplant with the oil.

3. Season generously with salt and pepper.

4. Spread the eggplant on the baking sheet and roast, turning once, until the eggplant is caramelized and tender, about 20 minutes.

5. Transfer the eggplant to a serving bowl and toss with the vinegar.

6. Top with the goat cheese and basil, and serve immediately.

INGREDIENT TIP: *Look for small or medium-size vegetables that are shiny, smooth, and firm but not hard. Pay close attention to the stem as well; it should be mold free and green for freshness.*

Per Serving Calories: 154; Total Fat: 12g; Cholesterol: 15mg; Sodium: 110mg; Total Carbohydrates: 7g; Sugar: 4g; Fiber: 4g; Protein: 5g

Roasted Cinnamon Celery Root

CARBS PER SERVING: 22G

SERVES 4 / PREP TIME: 10 MINUTES / COOK TIME: 20 MINUTES

Celery root is a truly ugly vegetable, with long, hairy roots clotted with dirt and a dingy-looking, scaly skin. However, when you cut all that outer appearance off, you are left with a vegetable that is fresh-tasting and creamy-fleshed. Do not buy celery root that has any damp or mushy spots or one that feels lighter than it looks. This vegetable can be stored for up to six months in the refrigerator, but can dry out and become light and woody if kept too long.

2 celery roots (about 1 pound total), peeled and diced
1 teaspoon extra-virgin olive oil
1 teaspoon butter, melted
½ teaspoon ground cinnamon
Sea salt
Freshly ground black pepper

1. Preheat the oven to 350°F. Line a baking sheet with aluminum foil.

2. In a large bowl, toss the celery roots with the oil.

3. Transfer the roots to the baking sheet and roast until very tender, about 20 minutes.

4. Remove them from the oven and transfer to a bowl.

5. Add the butter and cinnamon to the bowl and use a potato masher to mash the roots until fluffy.

6. Season with salt and pepper. Serve warm.

NUTRITION TIP: *Celery root, also known as celeriac, is low in calories and a great source of vitamin K, iron, phosphorus, and calcium. The antioxidants in celery root can help fight several types of cancer, including colon cancer.*

Per Serving Calories: 117; Total Fat: 3g; Cholesterol: 3mg; Sodium: 299mg; Total Carbohydrates: 22g; Sugar: 4g; Fiber: 4g; Protein: 4g

Roasted Beets, Carrots, and Parsnips

CARBS PER SERVING: 27G

SERVES 4 / PREP TIME: 10 MINUTES / COOK TIME: 30 MINUTES

Beets come in an assortment of striking colors ranging from pale yellow to a deep, luscious reddish purple. All these colors combine well with orange carrots. Roasting root vegetables brings out their sweet, rich flavor, which is enhanced by a splash of apple cider vinegar. Try growing your own beets in the garden or window boxes on your patio for a truly sublime cooking experience—field to fork.

1 pound beets, peeled and quartered

½ pound carrots, peeled and cut into chunks

½ pound parsnips, peeled and cut into chunks

1 tablespoon extra-virgin olive oil

1 teaspoon apple cider vinegar

Sea salt

Freshly ground black pepper

1. Preheat the oven to 375°F. Line a baking tray with aluminum foil.

2. In a large bowl, toss the beets, carrots, and parsnips with the oil and vinegar until everything is well coated. Spread them out on the baking sheet.

3. Roast until the vegetables are tender and lightly caramelized, about 30 minutes.

4. Transfer the vegetables to a serving bowl, season with salt and pepper, and serve warm.

Per Serving Calories: 148; Total Fat: 4g; Cholesterol: 0mg; Sodium: 196mg; Total Carbohydrates: 27g; Sugar: 15g; Fiber: 6g; Protein: 3g

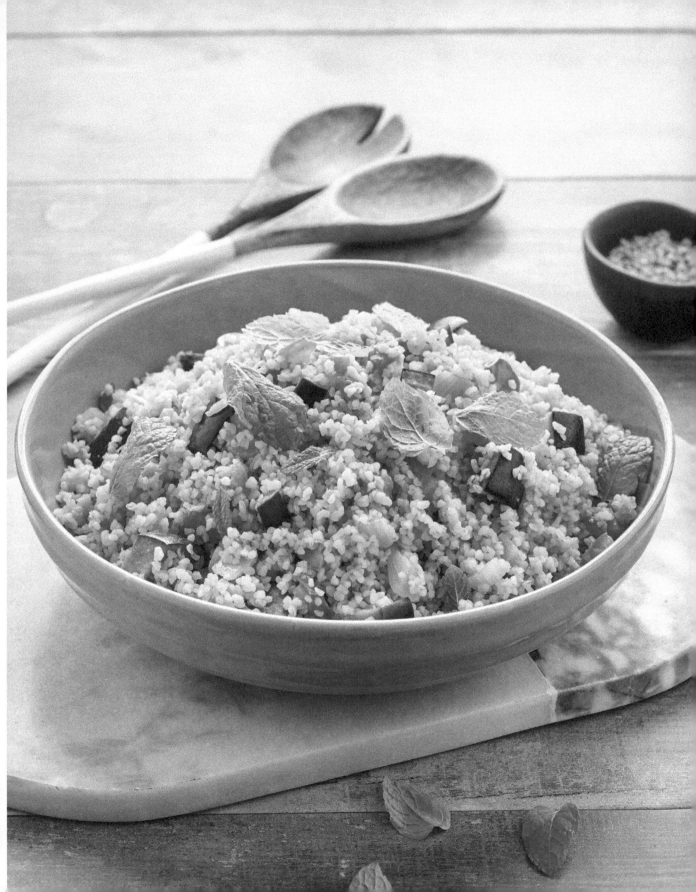

CHAPTER 10

Starch and Grain Sides

Mediterranean Chickpea Slaw

CARBS PER SERVING: 30G

SERVES 6 / PREP TIME: 10 MINUTES

Slaw is a traditional side for barbecue and a favorite potluck contribution. This version includes chickpeas and has a pleasing Greek-style dressing. Try to prepare this recipe ahead of time, to allow the balsamic vinegar to meld with the other ingredients. Just give the slaw a stir every hour or so to mix everything up, and wait until just before you serve it to sprinkle on the feta and parsley.

1 (15-ounce) can chickpeas packed in water, rinsed and drained
2 cups shredded kale
1 English cucumber, shredded
1 red bell pepper, seeded and cut into very thin strips
2 tablespoons balsamic vinegar
1 tablespoon chopped fresh oregano
Sea salt
Freshly ground black pepper
½ cup chopped fresh parsley
½ cup crumbled low-sodium feta cheese

1. In a large bowl, toss together the chickpeas, kale, cucumber, pepper, vinegar, and oregano.

2. Season with salt and pepper.

3. Sprinkle on the parsley and feta, and serve.

NUTRITION TIP: *If you are concerned about your sodium consumption, substitute soft goat cheese for the feta in this dish. This would cut the sodium by about 70mg per serving.*

Per Serving Calories: 192; Total Fat: 5g; Cholesterol: 8mg; Sodium: 168mg; Total Carbohydrates: 30g; Sugar: 6g; Fiber: 8g; Protein: 10g

Green Lentils with Olives and Summer Vegetables

CARBS PER SERVING: 49G

SERVES 4 / PREP TIME: 15 MINUTES

This fresh, filling dish could be a wonderful light lunch or a tasty side dish, depending on how hungry you are. Pine nuts add a surprising crunch and fresh chives a sharp taste that complement the buttery texture of the olives. The best way to chop your chives is to snip them with scissors, so you don't crush the stems.

3 tablespoons extra-virgin olive oil
2 tablespoons balsamic vinegar
2 teaspoons chopped fresh basil
1 teaspoon minced garlic
Sea salt
Freshly ground black pepper
2 (15-ounce) cans sodium-free green lentils, rinsed and drained
½ English cucumber, diced
2 tomatoes, diced
½ cup halved Kalamata olives
¼ cup chopped fresh chives
2 tablespoons pine nuts

1. Whisk together the olive oil, vinegar, basil, and garlic in a medium bowl. Season with salt and pepper.

2. Stir in the lentils, cucumber, tomatoes, olives, and chives.

3. Top with the pine nuts, and serve.

Per Serving Calories: 399; Total Fat: 15g; Cholesterol: 0mg; Sodium: 438mg; Total Carbohydrates: 49g; Sugar: 7g; Fiber: 19g; Protein: 20g

Sweet Potato Fennel Bake

CARBS PER SERVING: 33G

SERVES 4 / PREP TIME: 15 MINUTES / COOK TIME: 45 MINUTES

Sweet potato is often confused with or used interchangeably with yams, although they are very different vegetables. Sweet potatoes are part of the morning glory family, while yams are related to grasses; neither are actually potatoes. The orange tuber you are used to seeing in your local grocery store is probably a sweet potato. Sweet potatoes can have white, yellow, or orange flesh that is moist and sweet. Yams are starchier, drier, and have white or purplish flesh.

1 teaspoon butter
1 fennel bulb, trimmed
    and thinly sliced
2 sweet potatoes, peeled and
    thinly sliced
Freshly ground black pepper,
    to taste
½ teaspoon ground cinnamon
¼ teaspoon ground nutmeg
1 cup low-sodium
    vegetable broth

1. Preheat the oven to 375°F.

2. Lightly butter a 9-by-11-inch baking dish.

3. Arrange half the fennel in the bottom of the dish and top with half the sweet potatoes.

4. Season the potatoes with black pepper. Sprinkle half the cinnamon and nutmeg on the potatoes.

5. Repeat the layering to use up all the fennel, sweet potatoes, cinnamon, and nutmeg.

6. Pour in the vegetable broth and cover the dish with aluminum foil.

7. Bake until the vegetables are very tender, about 45 minutes.

8. Serve immediately.

Per Serving Calories: 153; Total Fat: 2g; Cholesterol: 2mg; Sodium: 178mg; Total Carbohydrates: 33g; Sugar: 1g; Fiber: 7g; Protein: 3g

Herbed Beans and Brown Rice

CARBS PER SERVING: 37G

SERVES 8 / PREP TIME: 15 MINUTES / COOK TIME: 15 MINUTES

Beans and rice is a traditional dish in many parts of the world. Both ingredients are very high in protein and iron, so the combination is a powerhouse of health benefits. Because the ingredients are relatively inexpensive yet provide important nutrition, families in many economically depressed areas of the world regularly eat meals based on them. Black beans, or any large, firm bean, can be used instead of the kidney beans.

2 teaspoons extra-virgin olive oil
½ sweet onion, chopped
1 teaspoon minced jalapeño pepper
1 teaspoon minced garlic
1 (15-ounce) can sodium-free red kidney beans, rinsed and drained
1 large tomato, chopped
1 teaspoon chopped fresh thyme
Sea salt
Freshly ground black pepper
2 cups cooked brown rice

1. Place a large skillet over medium-high heat and add the olive oil.

2. Sauté the onion, jalapeño, and garlic until softened, about 3 minutes.

3. Stir in the beans, tomato, and thyme.

4. Cook until heated through, about 10 minutes. Season with salt and pepper.

5. Serve over the warm brown rice.

SUBSTITUTION TIP: *If you have a little extra time, try boiling dried kidney beans for this dish instead of using canned. Soak them in cold water overnight, or put them in a bowl, cover with boiling water, and let them soak for an hour. Drain them and then just cover them with about 4 inches of fresh water and simmer until they're tender but not mushy, about 1 hour.*

Per Serving Calories: 199; Total Fat: 2g; Cholesterol: 0mg; Sodium: 37mg; Total Carbohydrates: 37g; Sugar: 2g; Fiber: 6g; Protein: 9g

Wild Rice with Blueberries and Pumpkin Seeds

CARBS PER SERVING: 37G

SERVES 4 / PREP TIME: 15 MINUTES / COOK TIME: 45 MINUTES

Wild rice is not a grain at all. It's a semi-aquatic grass that is indigenous to North America and is harvested in a way similar to the way rice is harvested in Asia—hence the name. Wild rice is high in protein, B vitamins, manganese, and dietary fiber. Unlike regular rice, you don't have to cook it until all the liquid is absorbed; you can boil a pot of water and simply drain off the excess when the rice is tender but still chewy, just as you would with pasta. This eliminates the chance of overcooking or burning the rice, which reduces stress in the kitchen.

1 tablespoon extra-virgin olive oil
½ sweet onion, chopped
2½ cups sodium-free chicken broth
1 cup wild rice, rinsed and drained
Pinch sea salt
½ cup toasted pumpkin seeds
½ cup blueberries
1 teaspoon chopped fresh basil

1. Place a medium saucepan over medium-high heat and add the oil.

2. Sauté the onion until softened and translucent, about 3 minutes.

3. Stir in the broth and bring to a boil.

4. Stir in the rice and salt and reduce the heat to low. Cover and simmer until the rice is tender, about 40 minutes.

5. Drain off any excess broth, if necessary. Stir in the pumpkin seeds, blueberries, and basil.

6. Serve warm.

NUTRITION TIP: *Blueberries have one of the highest antioxidant levels of any type of produce. If you can find only frozen blueberries for this dish, don't worry; the level of antioxidants does not drop, even after four months in the freezer.*

Per Serving Calories: 258; Total Fat: 9g; Cholesterol: 0mg; Sodium: 542mg; Total Carbohydrates: 37g; Sugar: 4g; Fiber: 4g; Protein: 11g

Mushroom Hazelnut Rice

CARBS PER SERVING: 39G

SERVES 8 / PREP TIME: 20 MINUTES / COOK TIME: 35 MINUTES

Hazelnuts, otherwise known as filberts, are extremely high in monounsaturated fatty acids, dietary fiber, vitamin E, and iron. Eating these sweet nuts can fight cancer, cut the risk of coronary disease, and support healthy bones. Mushrooms also contain iron, along with antioxidants, B vitamins, and vitamin D, so you have plenty of good reasons to give this tasty recipe a try.

1 tablespoon extra-virgin olive oil
1 cup chopped button mushrooms
½ sweet onion, chopped
1 celery stalk, chopped
2 teaspoons minced garlic
2 cups brown basmati rice
4 cups low-sodium chicken broth
1 teaspoon chopped fresh thyme
Sea salt
Freshly ground black pepper
½ cup chopped hazelnuts

1. Place a large saucepan over medium-high heat and add the oil.

2. Sauté the mushrooms, onion, celery, and garlic until lightly browned, about 10 minutes.

3. Add the rice and sauté for an additional minute.

4. Add the chicken broth and bring to a boil.

5. Reduce the heat to low and cover the pot. Simmer until the liquid is absorbed and the rice is tender, about 20 minutes.

6. Stir in the thyme and season with salt and pepper.

7. Top with the hazelnuts, and serve.

INGREDIENT TIP: *You can avoid any bitterness by removing the papery husk on the nut. Roast them for several minutes in a moderate oven and, after the nuts have cooled, rub the husks off between your palms.*

Per Serving Calories: 239; Total Fat: 6g; Cholesterol: 0mg; Sodium: 387mg; Total Carbohydrates: 39g; Sugar: 1g; Fiber: 1g; Protein: 7g

Barley Squash Risotto

CARBS PER SERVING: 32G

SERVES 6 / PREP TIME: 10 MINUTES / COOK TIME: 15 MINUTES

Don't panic when you see the word *risotto*, because you will not have to spend precious time stirring hot broth into Arborio rice for this dish. The grain is barley, and it is already cooked before you start sautéing your onion and garlic. The kale and squash are also previously cooked, which saves time and allows you to concentrate on other aspects of your meal. So next time you're cooking barley, kale, or butternut squash for another dish, make extra and you've got a future meal in the bag.

1 teaspoon extra-virgin olive oil

½ sweet onion, finely chopped

1 teaspoon minced garlic

2 cups cooked barley

2 cups chopped kale

2 cups cooked butternut squash, cut into ½-inch cubes

2 tablespoons chopped pistachios

1 tablespoon chopped fresh thyme

Sea salt

1. Place a large skillet over medium heat and add the oil.

2. Sauté the onion and garlic until softened and translucent, about 3 minutes.

3. Add the barley and kale, and stir until the grains are heated through and the greens are wilted, about 7 minutes.

4. Stir in the squash, pistachios, and thyme.

5. Cook until the dish is hot, about 4 minutes, and season with salt.

COOKING TIP: *Boiled squash will work in this dish, but if you want a rich, sweet flavor, roast the squash instead. Check it frequently to ensure it isn't overcooked and mushy.*

Per Serving Calories: 159; Total Fat: 2g; Cholesterol: 0mg; Sodium: 62mg; Total Carbohydrates: 32g; Sugar: 2g; Fiber: 7g; Protein: 5g

Bulgur and Eggplant Pilaf

CARBS PER SERVING: 54G

SERVES 4 / PREP TIME: 10 MINUTES / COOK TIME: 1 HOUR

Pilaf in its simplest form is just grain, usually rice, cooked in some sort of broth rather than water. In this case, the grain is bulgur and the liquid is chicken broth. Pilaf is very popular in Middle Eastern countries as well as Asia, South America, and the Caribbean. Pilaf can include meats, seafood, vegetables, herbs, and spices, depending on the region and culinary traditions.

1 tablespoon extra-virgin olive oil
½ sweet onion, chopped
2 teaspoons minced garlic
1 cup chopped eggplant
1½ cups bulgur
4 cups low-sodium chicken broth
1 cup diced tomato
Sea salt
Freshly ground black pepper
2 tablespoons chopped fresh basil

1. Place a large saucepan over medium-high heat. Add the oil and sauté the onion and garlic until softened and translucent, about 3 minutes.

2. Stir in the eggplant and sauté 4 minutes to soften.

3. Stir in the bulgur, broth, and tomatoes. Bring the mixture to a boil.

4. Reduce the heat to low, cover, and simmer until the water has been absorbed, about 50 minutes.

5. Season the pilaf with salt and pepper.

6. Garnish with the basil, and serve.

Per Serving Calories: 297; Total Fat: 4g; Cholesterol: 7mg; Sodium: 357mg; Total Carbohydrates: 54g; Sugar: 7g; Fiber: 12g; Protein: 14g

Whole-Wheat Couscous with Pecans

CARBS PER SERVING: 30G

SERVES 6 / PREP TIME: 10 MINUTES / COOK TIME: 5 MINUTES

Couscous looks like a grain but is actually pasta. Preparing couscous is one of the easiest cooking tasks you will ever undertake. Simply add boiling liquid to the couscous, cover, let it sit for about five minutes, and fluff with a fork. It is so simple that you might find yourself adding this delicious ingredient to many meals. This dish is actually more of a salad than a side dish because of the cold dressing, but it pairs well with almost every main course protein. Eat it in side dish amounts because it is relatively high in carbs.

FOR THE DRESSING
¼ cup extra-virgin olive oil
2 tablespoons
    balsamic vinegar
1 teaspoon honey
Sea salt
Freshly ground black pepper

FOR THE COUSCOUS
1¼ cups whole-
    wheat couscous
Pinch sea salt
1 teaspoon butter
2 cups boiling water
1 scallion, white and green
    parts, chopped
½ cup chopped pecans
2 tablespoons chopped
    fresh parsley

TO MAKE THE DRESSING

1. Whisk together the oil, vinegar, and honey.

2. Season with salt and pepper and set it aside.

TO MAKE THE COUSCOUS

1. Put the couscous, salt, and butter in a large heat-proof bowl and pour the boiling water on top. Stir and cover the bowl. Let it sit for 5 minutes. Uncover and fluff the couscous with a fork.

2. Stir in the dressing, scallion, pecans, and parsley.

3. Serve warm.

INGREDIENT TIP: *The best couscous for this side is Israeli couscous, which has larger grains and is visually appealing. You can find many types of couscous in your local grocery store, so choose the one that suits your palate.*

Per Serving Calories: 251; Total Fat: 13g; Cholesterol: 2mg; Sodium: 76mg; Total Carbohydrates: 30g; Sugar: 1g; Fiber: 2g; Protein: 5g

Quinoa Vegetable Skillet

CARBS PER SERVING: 26G

SERVES 6 / PREP TIME: 15 MINUTES / COOK TIME: 15 MINUTES

You are probably familiar with quinoa because it is one of the more trendy grain choices, especially with those looking to eat more healthily. Quinoa is very high in protein, fiber, calcium, and iron. This tasty ingredient is actually a complete protein, meaning it contains all eight essential amino acids, making it a popular item for vegetarians. There are several kinds of quinoa, so try a few to ensure you cook up your favorite.

2 cups vegetable broth
1 cup quinoa, well rinsed
    and drained
1 teaspoon extra-virgin
    olive oil
½ sweet onion, chopped
2 teaspoons minced garlic
½ large green zucchini, halved
    lengthwise and cut into
    half disks
1 red bell pepper, seeded and
    cut into thin strips
1 cup fresh or frozen
    corn kernels
1 teaspoon chopped
    fresh basil
Sea salt
Freshly ground black pepper

1. Place a medium saucepan over medium heat and add the vegetable broth. Bring the broth to a boil and add the quinoa. Cover and reduce the heat to low.

2. Cook until the quinoa has absorbed all the broth, about 15 minutes. Remove from the heat and let it cool slightly.

3. While the quinoa is cooking, place a large skillet over medium-high heat and add the oil.

4. Sauté the onion and garlic until softened and translucent, about 3 minutes.

5. Add the zucchini, bell pepper, and corn, and sauté until the vegetables are tender-crisp, about 5 minutes.

6. Remove the skillet from the heat. Add the cooked quinoa and the basil to the skillet, stirring to combine. Season with salt and pepper, and serve.

Per Serving Calories: 158; Total Fat: 3g; Cholesterol: 0mg; Sodium: 298mg; Total Carbohydrates: 26g; Sugar: 3g; Fiber: 3g; Protein: 7g

Coconut Quinoa

CARBS PER SERVING: 35G

SERVES 4 / PREP TIME: 15 MINUTES / COOK TIME: 25 MINUTES

Coconut milk creates a creamy side dish that might remind you of rice pudding in appearance but certainly won't in taste. Sweet onion or Vidalia onion is preferable to harsher white or Spanish onions here, and you probably will not cry as much while cutting the milder varieties. You can pair this quinoa with grilled chicken breasts or spiced shrimp skewers for a lovely, filling meal. Top the dish with a scattering of chopped fresh cilantro for a pretty presentation.

2 teaspoons extra-virgin olive oil

1 sweet onion, chopped

1 tablespoon grated fresh ginger

2 teaspoons minced garlic

1 cup low-sodium chicken broth

1 cup coconut milk

1 cup quinoa, well rinsed and drained

Sea salt

¼ cup shredded, unsweetened coconut

1. Place a large saucepan over medium-high heat and add the oil.

2. Sauté the onion, ginger, and garlic until softened, about 3 minutes.

3. Add the chicken broth, coconut milk, and quinoa.

4. Bring the mixture to a boil, then reduce the heat to low and cover. Simmer the quinoa, stirring occasionally, until the quinoa is tender and most of the liquid has been absorbed, about 20 minutes.

5. Season the quinoa with salt, and serve topped with the coconut.

Per Serving Calories: 354; Total Fat: 21g; Cholesterol: 0mg; Sodium: 32mg; Total Carbohydrates: 35g; Sugar: 4g; Fiber: 6g; Protein: 9g

Whole-Wheat Linguine with Kale Pesto

CARBS PER SERVING: 25G

SERVES 6 / PREP TIME: 10 MINUTES / COOK TIME: 20 MINUTES

Pasta is often a course by itself in a larger meal, rather than an accompaniment, and this glorious rich dish would be perfect that way. But you can have it as a small side to cut down on the carbs. Sun-dried tomatoes are a stunning addition to the pesto, adding color and richness. Use oil-packed sun-dried tomatoes rather than dried ones, or you will have to reconstitute the tomatoes in water before using them.

½ cup shredded kale
½ cup fresh basil
½ cup sun-dried tomatoes
¼ cup chopped almonds
2 tablespoons extra-virgin olive oil
8 ounces dry whole-wheat linguine
½ cup grated Parmesan cheese

1. Place the kale, basil, sun-dried tomatoes, almonds, and olive oil in a food processor or blender, and pulse until a chunky paste forms, about 2 minutes. Scoop the pesto into a bowl and set it aside.

2. Place a large pot filled with water on high heat and bring to a boil.

3. Cook the pasta al dente, according to the package directions.

4. Drain the pasta and toss it with the pesto and the Parmesan cheese.

5. Serve immediately.

NUTRITION TIP: *Basil is a stellar source of vitamin K and disease-fighting flavonoids. It supports the cardiovascular system and helps slow the progression of conditions such as rheumatoid arthritis.*

Per Serving Calories: 217; Total Fat: 10g; Cholesterol: 34mg; Sodium: 194mg; Total Carbohydrates: 25g; Sugar: 2g; Fiber: 1g; Protein: 9g

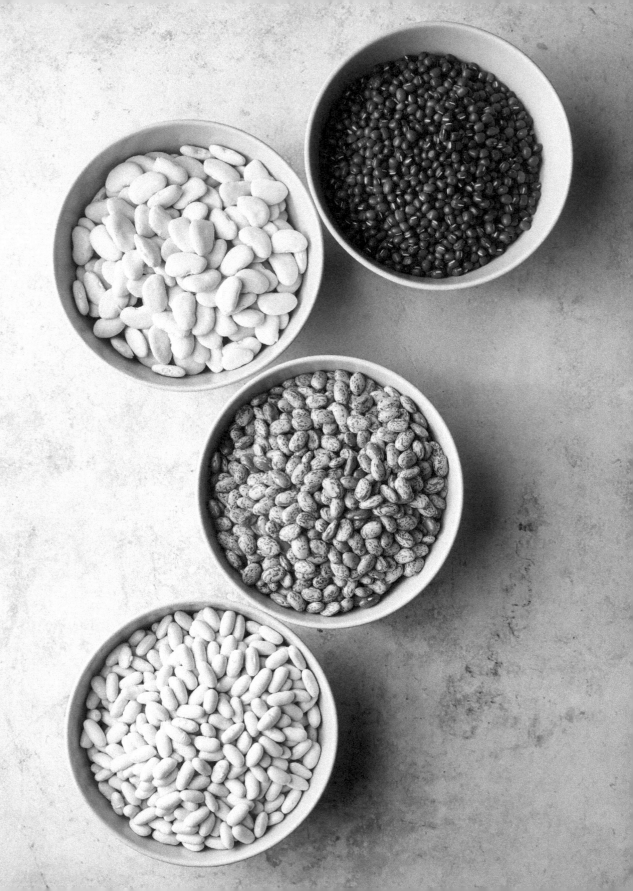

RESOURCES

Activity Trackers

Activity trackers help people achieve their activity goals. Their functions run the gamut, from tracking steps and calories to monitoring sleep and heart rate. Find one that suits your needs. There are four popular activity trackers.

- Fitbit, www.fitbit.com
- Garmin Vivofit, explore.garmin.com/en-US/vivo-fitness/
- Jawbone, jawbone.com
- Withings Go, www.withings.com/us/en/products/withings-go

Calorie-Counting Websites

- **Calorie King** (www.calorieking.com) This site has a large database of nutrients found in foods, including calories, carbohydrates, fiber, fat, and protein.
- **United States Department of Agriculture (USDA) Food Composition Database** (ndb.nal.usda.gov/ndb/search/list) This is the gold standard for tracking the nutrient composition of foods.

Calorie-Tracking Apps

Studies have shown that people who track what they eat can lose up to 50 percent more weight. Both of these apps also track nutrients like carbohydrates, sodium, fat, and protein.

- **Lose It!** This is another easy-to-use free calorie and activity tracker. It also has an active chat community and offers you the ability to participate in challenges.
- **Myfitnesspal.com** This is one of the most popular calorie counters. Based on your weight, height, age, and goals, it will make recommendations on how many calories you should eat a day. It can also sync with a fitness tracking device, like Fitbit. It has a huge database and will even scan bar codes of some packaged foods. It is free.

Exercise

♦ **American Council on Exercise** has exercise videos for every fitness level at www.acefitness.org/acefit/exercise-library-main/. You'll also find articles on exercising with diabetes at www.acefitness.org/acefit/search_results. aspx?searchsite=consumer&searchstring=diabetes.

♦ The **Office of Disease Prevention and Health Promotion** (Health.gov) has a free downloadable booklet with tips on physical activity called "Physical Activity Guidelines for Americans." You can get it at health.gov/paguidelines/guidelines/.

Find Health Professionals

♦ A **Certified Diabetes Educator** (CDE) is a health professional who has comprehensive knowledge of and experience in diabetes management, prediabetes, and diabetes prevention. Find a CDE at www.ncbde.org/find-a-cde/.

♦ A **Registered Dietitian** (RD) is a trained nutrition professional who has met the strict educational and experiential standards set forth by the Commission on Dietetic Registration (CDR) of the Academy of Nutrition and Dietetics (AND). Find an RD at www.eatright.org/find-an-expert.

♦ The **American Council on Exercise** (ACE) certifies fitness professionals who promote safe and effective physical activity. Find an ACE-certified fitness trainer at www.acefitness.org/acefit/locate-trainer/.

Meditation Apps

Meditation is one of the best ways to combat stress. This is especially important for people with diabetes, because stress can raise blood sugar. Here are a few meditation apps you can download and take with you anywhere.

♦ Buddhify, buddhify.com

♦ Headspace, www.headspace.com

♦ Calm, www.calm.com

Websites for Diabetes Information

♦ *American Diabetes Association (diabetes.org)* is a national organization for health professionals and people with diabetes that provides useful information about living well and managing type 2 diabetes.

♦ *American Heart Association (americanheart.org)* is the nation's oldest and largest voluntary organization dedicated to fighting heart disease and stroke. It provides helpful information on diet, exercise, stress management, and healthy living for health professionals and consumers.

♦ *Academy of Nutrition and Dietetics (eatright.org)* is a national organization for registered dietitians in the United States and is the most credible source of nutrition information.

♦ *dLife.com (www.dlife.com)* offers a wealth of information to give you the answers you need to manage your diabetes health. They have a large collection of diabetes videos on topics ranging from cooking to exercise.

♦ *Joslin Diabetes Center (joslin.harvard.edu)* is world-renowned for its expertise in diabetes treatment and research. It has useful information for health professionals and people with diabetes.

REFERENCES

Academy of Nutrition and Dietetics. "Position Statement of the Academy of Nutrition and Dietetics: Use of Nutritive and Non-Nutritive Sweeteners." May 2012. Accessed October 25, 2016. www.eatrightpro.org/resource/practice/position-and-practice -papers/position-papers/use-of-nutritive-and-nonnutritive-sweeteners

American College of Sports Medicine. "Exercise and Type 2 Diabetes: American College of Sports Medicine and the American Diabetes Association: Joint Position Statement." December 2010. Accessed November 8, 2016. www.ncbi.nlm.nih.gov/pmc/articles /PMC2992225/

American Diabetes Association. "Alcohol." June 6, 2014. Accessed October 20, 2016. www.diabetes.org/food-and-fitness/food/what-can-i-eat/making-healthy-food -choices/alcohol.html.

American Diabetes Association. "Exercise Can Help Tame Type 2 Diabetes, Say New Guidelines." December 9, 2010. Accessed October 24, 2016. www.diabetes.org/newsroom /press-releases/2010/exercise-can-help-tame-type-2.ht ml.

American Diabetes Association. "Physical Activity/Exercise and Diabetes: A Position Statement of the American Diabetes Association." November 2016. Accessed December 19, 2016. http://care.diabetesjournals.org/content/39/11/2065

American Diabetes Association. "Standards of Medical Care in Diabetes—2016." January 2016. Accessed October 25, 2016. care.diabetesjournals.org/content/suppl/2015/12/21 /39.Supplement_1.DC2/2016-Standards-of-Care.pdf.

American Diabetes Association. "What We Recommend." May 19, 2015. Accessed October 24, 2016. www.diabetes.org/food-and-fitness/fitness/types-of-activity /what-we-recommend.html.

American Heart Association. "The American Heart Association's Diet and Lifestyle Recommendations." October 24, 2016. Accessed October 24, 2016. www.heart.org /HEARTORG/HealthyLiving/HealthyEating/Nutrition/The-American-Heart -Associations-Diet-and-Lifestyle-Recommendations_UCM_305855_Article.jsp# .WA7FHIWcGUk.

Centers for Disease Control and Prevention. "Diabetes Report Card 2014." Accessed October 24, 2016. www.cdc.gov/diabetes/pdfs/library/diabetesreportcard2014.pdf.

Centers for Disease Control and Prevention. "Number of Americans with Diabetes Projected to Double or Triple by 2050." October 22, 2010. Accessed October 24, 2016. www.cdc.gov/media/pressrel/2010/r101022.html.

Centers for Disease Control and Prevention. "Press Release: One in Five Adults Meet Overall Physical Activity Guidelines." May 2, 2013. Accessed October 24, 2016. www.cdc.gov/media/releases/2013/p0502-physical-activity.html.

2015–2020 Dietary Guidelines for Americans. 8th Edition. "Appendix 2. Estimated Calorie Needs per Day, by Age, Sex, and Physical Activity Level." Accessed October 24, 2016. health.gov/dietaryguidelines/2015/guidelines/appendix-2/.

2015–2020 Dietary Guidelines for Americans. 8th Edition. "Key Recommendations: Components of Healthy Eating Patterns." Accessed October 24, 2016. health.gov/dietaryguidelines/2015/guidelines/chapter-1/key-recommendations/.

Harvard School of Public Health. "Artificial Sweeteners." Accessed October 25, 2016. www.hsph.harvard.edu/nutritionsource/healthy-drinks/artificial-sweeteners/.

Kaiser Permanente. "Kaiser Permanente Study Finds Keeping a Food Diary Doubles Diet Weight Loss." July 8, 2008. Accessed October 24, 2016. share.kaiserpermanente.org/article/kaiser-permanente-study-finds-keeping-a-food-diary-doubles-diet-weight-loss/.

Medicine & Science in Sports & Exercise. "Exercise and Type 2 Diabetes: American College of Sports Medicine and the American Diabetes Association: Joint Position Statement." December 2010. Accessed October 24, 2016. journals.lww.com/acsm-msse/Fulltext/2010/12000/Exercise_and_Type_2_Diabetes__American_College_of.18.aspx.

National Institute of Diabetes and Digestive and Kidney Diseases. "Diabetes Prevention Program (DPP)." Accessed October 24, 2016. www.niddk.nih.gov/about-niddk/research-areas/diabetes/diabetes-prevention-program-dpp/Pages/default.aspx.

National Sleep Foundation. "Healthy Sleep Tips." Accessed October 24, 2016. sleepfoundation.org/sleep-tools-tips/healthy-sleep-tips.

Pastors, Joyce Green, Marilyn S. Arnold, Anne Daly, Marion Franz, and Hope S. Warshaw. *Diabetes Nutrition Q&A for Health Professionals: 101 Essential Questions Answered by Experts.* Alexandria, VA: American Diabetes Association, 2003.

U.S. Department of Health and Human Services. *"2008 Physical Activity Guidelines for Americans*: Summary." Accessed October 24, 2016. health.gov/paguidelines/guidelines/summary.aspx.

Wansink, Brian. *Mindless Eating—Why We Eat More Than We Think.* New York: Bantam-Dell, 2006.

WebMD. "Diabetes Epidemic Will Hit Half of U.S. by 2020." November 23, 2010. Accessed October 24, 2016. www.webmd.com/diabetes/news/20101123/diabetes-epidemic-will-hit-half-of-us-by-2020#1.

Young, Lisa R., and Marion Nestle. "Expanding Portion Sizes in the US Marketplace: Implications for Nutrition Counseling." *Journal of the American Dietetic Association* 100, no. 2 (February 2003): 232–234. portionteller.com/pdf/portsize.pdf.

GLYCEMIC INDEX AND GLYCEMIC LOAD FOOD LISTS

The following is a list of the glycemic index and glycemic load of many common carbohydrates. Foods are ranked between 0 and 100 based on how they affect one's blood glucose level. The best choices are low glycemic, which have a rating of 55 or less, and medium glycemic, which have a rating of 56 to 69.

Remember that it is more important to pay attention to the glycemic load of a food, that is, the amount of carbohydrates it contains per serving. The best choices have low (less than 10) or moderate (between 10 and 20) loads.

GLYCEMIC INDEX AND GLYCEMIC LOAD OF COMMON FOODS

FOOD	GLYCEMIC INDEX	SERVING SIZE (GRAMS)	GLYCEMIC LOAD (PER SERVING)
BAKERY PRODUCTS			
Bagel, white	72	70	25
Baguette, white	95	30	15
Barley bread	34	30	7
Corn tortilla	52	50	12
Croissant	67	57	17
Doughnut	76	47	17
Pita bread	68	30	10
Sourdough rye	48	30	6
Soya and linseed bread	36	30	3
Sponge cake	46	63	17
Wheat tortilla	30	50	8
White wheat flour bread	71	30	10
Whole-wheat bread	71	30	9

FOOD	GLYCEMIC INDEX	SERVING SIZE (GRAMS)	GLYCEMIC LOAD (PER SERVING)
BEVERAGES			
Apple juice, unsweetened	44	250mL	30
Coca-Cola	63	250mL	16
Gatorade	78	250mL	12
Lucozade	95	250mL	40
Orange juice, unsweetened	50	250mL	12
Tomato juice, canned	38	250mL	4
BREAKFAST CEREALS			
All-Bran	55	30	12
Coco Pops	77	30	20
Cornflakes	93	30	23
Muesli	66	30	16
Oatmeal	55	50	13
Special K	69	30	14
DAIRY			
Ice cream, regular	57	50	6
Milk, full fat	41	250 mL	5
Milk, skim	32	250 mL	4
Reduced-fat yogurt with fruit	33	200	11
FRUITS			
Apple	39	120	6
Banana, ripe	62	120	16
Cherries	22	120	3
Dates, dried	42	60	18
Grapefruit	25	120	3
Grapes	59	120	11
Mango	41	120	8
Orange	40	120	4

FOOD	GLYCEMIC INDEX	SERVING SIZE (GRAMS)	GLYCEMIC LOAD (PER SERVING)
Peach	42	120	5
Pear	38	120	4
Pineapple	51	120	8
Raisins	64	60	28
Strawberries	40	120	1
Watermelon	72	120	4
GRAINS			
Brown rice	50	150	16
Buckwheat	45	150	13
Bulgur	30	50	11
Corn on the cob	60	150	20
Couscous	65	150	9
Fettucini	32	180	15
Gnocchi	68	180	33
Macaroni	47	180	23
Quinoa	53	150	13
Spaghetti, white	46	180	22
Spaghetti, whole-wheat	42	180	26
Vermicelli	35	180	16
White rice	89	150	43
LEGUMES			
Baked beans	40	150	6
Black beans	30	150	7
Butter beans	36	150	8
Chickpeas	10	150	3
Kidney beans	29	150	7
Lentils	29	150	5
Navy beans	31	150	9
Soybeans	50	150	1

FOOD	GLYCEMIC INDEX	SERVING SIZE (GRAMS)	GLYCEMIC LOAD (PER SERVING)
SNACK FOODS			
Cashews, salted	27	50	3
Corn chips, salted	42	50	11
Fruit Roll-Ups	99	30	24
Graham crackers	74	25	14
Honey	61	25	12
Hummus	6	30	0
M&M's, peanut	33	30	6
Microwave popcorn, plain	55	20	6
Muesli bar	61	30	13
Nutella	33	20	4
Peanuts	7	50	0
Potato chips	51	50	12
Pretzels	83	30	16
Rice cakes	82	25	17
Rye crisps	64	25	11
Shortbread	64	25	10
Vanilla wafers	77	25	14
VEGETABLES			
Beetroot	64	80	4
Carrot	35	80	2
Green peas	51	80	4
Parsnip	52	80	4
Sweet potato	70	150	22
White potato, boiled	81	150	22
Yam	54	150	20

Sources: Harvard Health Publications (http://www.health.harvard.edu/healthy-eating/glycemic_index_and_glycemic_load_for_100_foods) and Mendosa.com (http://www.mendosa.com/gilists.htm).

CARBOHYDRATE AND CALORIE VALUES

Understanding the carbohydrate and calorie content of common foods can help you plan your meals. These values are derived from NutritionData.com, which is a useful site for calculating nutritional information.

BREADS, CEREALS, & PASTAS

Each of the serving sizes listed below offers 15g carbs

Bread, white or whole wheat, pumpernickel, rye (1 slice or 1 oz); 65 cals

Bun, hamburger/hot dog (½ bun or 1 oz), 80 cals

Crackers, Saltine or round butter (4 to 6); 70 cals

English muffin (½); 65 cals

Melba toast (4 slices); 60 cals

Oyster crackers (20); 100 cals

Tortilla, corn or flour (6 inches across); 60 cals

Barley, cooked (⅓ cup); 70 cals

Couscous, cooked (⅓ cup); 60 cals

Pasta, cooked (⅓ cup); 75 cals

Quinoa, cooked (½ cup), 70 cals

Rice, white or brown, cooked (⅓ cup); 70 cals

STARCHY VEGETABLES

Each of the serving sizes listed below offers 15g carbs

Butternut squash, cooked (¾ cup); 75 cals

Corn (½ cup); 65 cals

Potato, baked (1 small or ¼ large, 3 oz); 57 cals

Pumpkin, cooked (1 cup small cubes); 50 cals

Sweet potato (½ cup); 54 cals

BEANS & LENTILS

Each of the serving sizes listed below offers 12–15g carbs

Baked beans (¼ cup); 60 cals

Black beans, cooked (¼ cup); 70 cals

Garbanzo beans, cooked (¼ cup); 90 cals

Kidney beans, cooked (¼ cup); 70 cals

Navy beans, cooked (¼ cup); 80 cals

Lima beans, cooked (¼ cup); 64 cals

Pinto beans, cooked (¼ cup); 80 cals

BEANS & LENTILS *continued*

White beans cooked (¼ cup); 80 cals

Hummus (⅓ cup); 135 cals

Lentils, cooked (½ cup); 64 cals

Peas—black-eyed, split, cooked (½ cup);

Refried beans (½ cup)

NONSTARCHY VEGETABLES

*Each of the serving sizes
listed below offers 15g carbs*

Beets, cooked (1 cup); 74 cals

Broccoli, cooked (1 cup chopped); 44 cals

Brussels sprouts, cooked (1 cup); 56 cals

Cabbage, raw (2 cups); 56 cals

Carrots, (1 cup); 70 cals

Cauliflower, raw (3 cups); 75 cals

Celery, raw (5 cups, chopped); 80 cals

Chard, raw (15 cups); 105 cals

Cucumber, raw (5 cups); 80 cals

Eggplant, raw (3 cups); 60.cals

Green beans, raw (2 cups); 70 cals

Kale, raw (2 cups); 66 cals

Okra, cooked (3 cups); 54 cals

Radishes, raw (3 cups); 57 cals

Romaine lettuce, shredded (6 cups); 48 cals

Spinach, raw (15 cups); 105 cals

Tomatoes, raw (2 cups); 54 cals

Zucchini, raw (3 cups); 60 cals

FRUIT

*Each of the serving sizes
listed below offers 15g carbs*

Apple (¾ cup, chopped); 60 cals

Apricots, raw (¾ cup); 65 cals

Banana (½ cup); 67 cals

Blueberries (¾ cup); 63 cals

Cantaloupe (1 cup cubes); 60 cals

Cherries (12); 60 cals

Grapefruit, large (½); 52 cals

Grapes (1 cup); 62 cals

Kiwi (1); 56 cals

Mango (½ cup); 53 cals

Orange (1 small); 65 cals

Papaya (1 cup cubes); 55 cals

Peach (1 medium); 59 cals

Pear (½ large); 66 cals

Pineapple (¾ cup); 63 cals

Plum (2 small); 60 cals

Raspberries (1 cup; 64 cals

Strawberries (1 cup, sliced), 53 cals

Watermelon (1¼ cups, cubed), 57 cals

MILK

*Each of the serving sizes
listed below offers 12–15g carbs*

Low-fat plain yogurt (⅔ cup); 100 cals

Milk 2% (1 cup); 138 cals

MEASUREMENT CONVERSIONS

VOLUME EQUIVALENTS (DRY)

US STANDARD	METRIC (APPROXIMATE)
⅛ teaspoon	0.5 mL
¼ teaspoon	1 mL
½ teaspoon	2 mL
¾ teaspoon	4 mL
1 teaspoon	5 mL
1 tablespoon	15 mL
¼ cup	59 mL
⅓ cup	79 mL
½ cup	118 mL
⅔ cup	156 mL
¾ cup	177 mL
1 cup	235 mL
2 cups or 1 pint	475 mL
3 cups	700 mL
4 cups or 1 quart	1 L
½ gallon	2 L
1 gallon	4 L

VOLUME EQUIVALENTS (LIQUID)

US STANDARD	US STANDARD (OUNCES)	METRIC (APPROXIMATE)
2 tablespoons	1 fl. oz.	30 mL
¼ cup	2 fl. oz.	60 mL
½ cup	4 fl. oz.	120 mL
1 cup	8 fl. oz.	240 mL
1½ cups	12 fl. oz.	355 mL
2 cups or 1 pint	16 fl. oz.	475 mL
4 cups or 1 quart	32 fl. oz.	1 L
1 gallon	128 fl. oz.	4 L

OVEN TEMPERATURES

FAHRENHEIT (F)	CELSIUS (C) (APPROXIMATE)
250°F	120°C
300°F	150°C
325°F	165°C
350°F	180°C
375°F	190°C
400°F	200°C
425°F	220°C
450°F	230°C

THE DIRTY DOZEN AND CLEAN FIFTEEN

A nonprofit and environmental watchdog organization called Environmental Working Group (EWG) looks at data supplied by the US Department of Agriculture (USDA) and the Food and Drug Administration (FDA) about pesticide residues and compiles a list each year of the best and worst pesticide loads found in commercial crops. You can refer to the Dirty Dozen list to know which fruits and vegetables you should always buy organic. The Clean Fifteen list lets you know which produce is considered safe enough when grown conventionally to allow you to skip the organics. This does not mean that the Clean Fifteen produce is pesticide-free, though, so wash these fruits and vegetables thoroughly.

These lists change every year, so make sure you look up the most recent before you fill your shopping cart. You'll find the most recent lists as well as a guide to pesticides in produce at EWG.org/FoodNews.

2016 DIRTY DOZEN

Apples

Celery

Cherry tomatoes

Cucumbers

Grapes

Nectarines

Peaches

Potatoes

Snap peas

Spinach

Strawberries

Sweet bell peppers

In addition to the Dirty Dozen, the EWG added two foods contaminated with highly toxic organo-phosphate insecticides:

Hot peppers

Kale/Collard greens

2016 CLEAN FIFTEEN

Asparagus

Avocados

Cabbage

Cantaloupe

Cauliflower

Eggplant

Grapefruit

Kiwis

Mangoes

Onions

Papayas

Pineapples

Sweet corn

Sweet peas (frozen)

Sweet potatoes

RECIPE INDEX

INDEX

CPSIA information can be obtained
at www.ICGtesting.com
Printed in the USA
JSHW021422280919
1642JS00001B/1

9 781623 158330

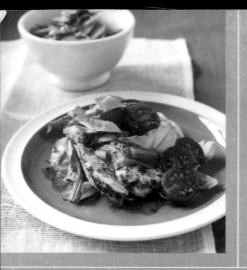
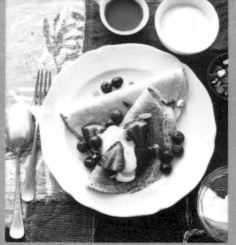
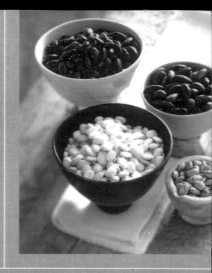

You CAN Eat and Live Well with Type 2 Diabetes

Receiving a type 2 diabetes diagnosis can be frightening—and learning to manage your diabetes through nutrition and lifestyle changes can feel overwhelming. But with *The Type 2 Diabetic Cookbook and Action Plan*, you can learn how to truly eat and live well. Registered dietitian and certified diabetes educator Martha McKittrick and cookbook author Michelle Anderson have combined their expertise to create this comprehensive, yet easy-to-follow resource for those with type 2 diabetes to learn about their management options, and implement a holistic, actionable, 3-month nutrition kick-starter right away.

- **FIND THE PLAN THAT'S RIGHT FOR YOU** with a fully customizable two-week meal plan with options for three different calorie-level needs

- **RETHINK YOUR FOOD** and discover how you can make the smartest food choices for your body's new nutritional needs

- **GET THE SUPPORT YOU NEED** to face day-to-day challenges so that you feel prepared and empowered no matter what comes your way

MARTHA MCKITTRICK, RDN, CDE is a registered dietitian, certified dietitian–nutritionist and certified diabetes educator in New York City. She specializes in weight control, cardiovascular health, diabetes, sports nutrition, PCOS, GI issues including IBS, women's health and preventive nutrition. Martha has helped hundreds of patients understand exactly what they need to do to manage their type 2 diabetes through diet, exercise, and self care.

MICHELLE ANDERSON is a writer, chef, and recipe developer, who specializes in medically restricted diets. She has written numerous cookbooks on a variety of subject matter such as PCOS, autoimmune paleo protocol, and insulin resistance, as well as holistic health.

COOKING / DIET U.S. $15.99
ISBN 978-1-62315-833-0
51599>

9 781623 158330

WWW.ROCKRIDGEPRESS.COM